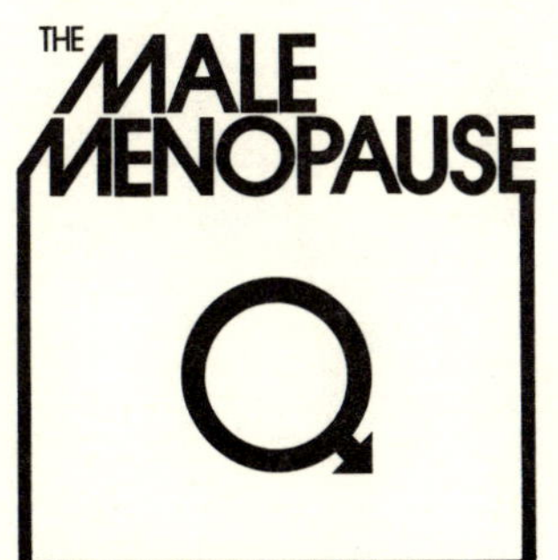

THE MALE MENOPAUSE

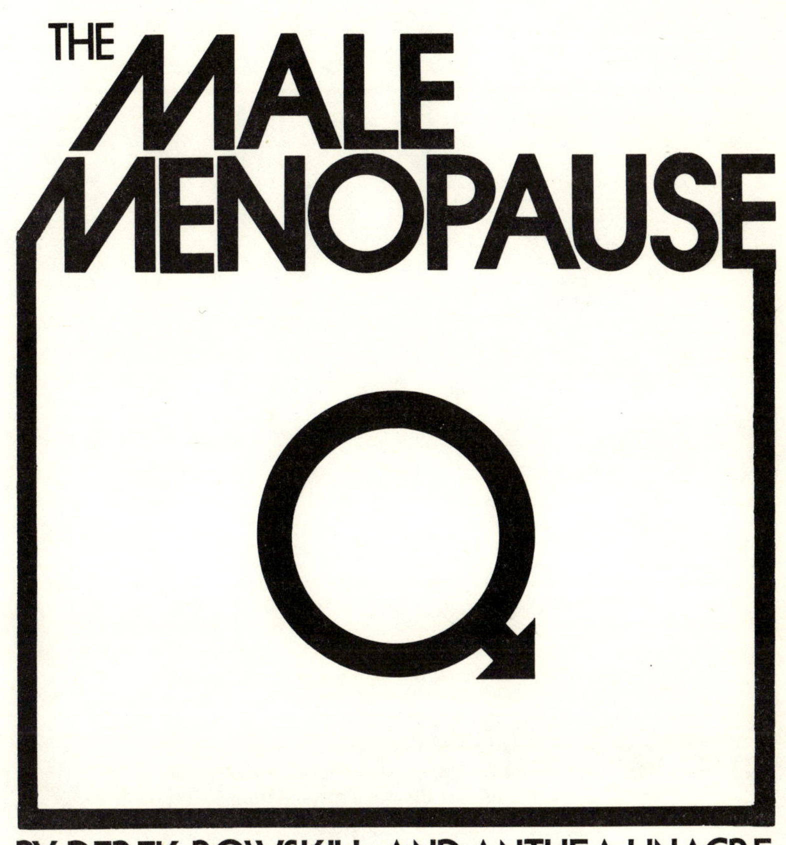

BY DEREK BOWSKILL AND ANTHEA LINACRE

Foreword by Robert Chartham

BROOKE HOUSE PUBLISHERS
LOS ANGELES

Printed and bound in Great Britain

Library of Congress Cataloging in Publication Data

Bowskill, Derek.
    The "male" menopause.

    Bibliography: p.
    1. Climacteric, Male.   I. Linacre, Anthea,
joint author.   II. Title.
RC884.B67   616.6′93   76-30659
ISBN 0-912588-15-2

Contents

Acknowledgements

We gratefully acknowledge the willing help given to us by the many un-named contributors to our book. We would also like to thank the following for their valuable assistance and advice:

Dr. John Bancroft — M.D.,M.R.C.P.,F.R.C., Psych Clinical Reader in Psychiatry

Dr. Michael Bott — Consultant Psychiatrist

John Bratby R.A.

Tony Britton

Surgeon Vice-Admiral Sir Dick Caldwell, K.B.E.,C.B.,M.D., F.R.C.P. (Ed) F.R.C.P. (Lond.)

Quentin Crisp — Author of 'How to Have a Life Style' and 'The Naked Civil Servant'

Dr. David Delvin — Medical Editor of 'General Practitioner'

Dr. Dennis Friedman — Of the Dept. of Psychological Medicine, St. Bartholomew's Hospital, London

Dr. James Hemming — Psychologist, author, lecturer and counsellor

J. Ellsworth Laing — Of the Wessex Centre for Plastic and Maxillo-Facial Surgery

Joan Mackay

Richard Price — Co-director, Phyllis Wright (Health and Hygiene) Ltd. Marital-Aids Specialists of Croydon, Surrey

Claire and Des Rayner

Paul Rimmer — Founder of the first English company to deal in sex-aids (1967)

Dr. Peter Scales — M.R.C.S.,L.R.C.P.,D.L.O. Principal in general practice, who for the past twenty years has taken a special interest in the problems and counselling of sexual dysfunctions

Dr. Robert Sharpe — Founder of the Institute of Behaviour Therapy

Dr. Prudence Tunnadine — Training Secretary of the Institute of Psycho-Sexual Medicine

Sidney Wasserman   M.S.S.A.,D.W.S., Casework Consultant to the Social Services. Former Associate Professor of Social Work, Smith College School of Social Work, Northampton, Mass., U.S.A. and Lecturer,University of Bradford, Bradford, England.

Colin Wilson   For his special contribution, and the extract from his book 'Mysteries'.

We apologise for any errors.

Preface

Strange events overtake some men in the middle of life. Paul Gauguin and Albert Schweitzer are but two.

Gauguin was 43 when he forsook established business life in Paris to take up painting in the South Seas. Schweitzer was 38 when he renounced fame and fortune as a brilliant exponent of Bach to start his chicken-coop hospital in Lambarene.

There comes a time in most men's lives when they feel a need to re-assess who they are and what is happening to them; to re-evaluate their priorities; and to re-examine their achievements in the light of their hopes, dreams and expectations. Many find themselves at odds with their cherished self-images. Sometimes the discovery may grow over four or five years, and sometimes it descends like a religious conversion.

In the past, this process has had many names: mid-life identity crisis; middle-age anxiety; involutional melancholia; metabolic depression; and the climacteric. Now it has attracted a new name: The *'male' menopause* . . . and there are few men — and hardly any women — who do not accept this paradoxical description as valid.

During our research, it became clear that this title was not just a handy phrase for something quite other; not just media jargon; nor was it quasi, spurious or counterfeit. In fact, the nomenclature suits the condition perfectly: the MM is absurd, irrational and paradoxical.

The man is no longer in control of what is happening to him. His unconscious — perhaps after a life-time of frustration — is moving around, trying to find an opening. The Kraken of his Psyche has wakened and started to rebel. Generally, the man will respond in one of two ways: he will inflate or deflate . . . implode or explode; in his own eyes a Don Juan or a Don Quixote, but in society's, an ageing hippy with neither the success and magnetism of the first nor the idealism and chivalry of the second . . . a ridiculous anachronism — premature, immature and generally mal à propos.

However, the victims are among the most wretched of us . . . deserving only compassion but unable to accept it because of their self-defeating mannerisms and their self-perpetuating mechanisms. But, awareness itself being therapeutic, we hope this book will illuminate and ameliorate the strangely disturbing syndrome; for, without foresight and insight, there is no doubt that the *'male' menopause* can be a disastrous watershed for Twentieth Century Man.

Personal Note

I am 47: neither too young nor too old to be out of range of the fire, the 'foolish fire', of the 'male' menopause; and there are very few of the symptoms described in the book that I have not experienced at one time or another and in all kinds of combinations and permutations. Like J. Alfred Prufrock,

> "I have known them all already, known them all
> Have known the evenings, mornings, afternoons,
> I have measured out my life with coffee spoons."

And not only coffee spoons; many others too — some quite greasy and dirty.

From my own not always secure grip upon the human condition I have come to realise that the problem is simply one of arithmetic. If you add up your life's symptoms incorrectly, you become fair game for mania or depression . . . or the malaise of our time, the 'male' menopause. And we are no more than the sum of our parts. We are who we are.

Estragon has a line in *Waiting for Godot,* "Nothing to be done". I judge that sentiment to be wrong. I suggest there is everything to be done — and what is more important, that anyone can do it. Anybody can do anything. It is only the manipulators and the protectors of the status quo who will tell you otherwise. Anybody can do anything — so you can choose. If you are a man, you can choose to have the 'male' menopause — and you can choose not to have it. I doubt neither its existence nor its impact — nor do I doubt your ability and privilege to reject it. The choice is yours. You can scorn and spurn it at will.

I hope this book helps you to do so.

Derek Bowskill, London, March 1976

Personal Note

Aptly enough, it was while being chatted up by a middle-aged executive, that the idea of writing a book on the *'male'* *menopause* arose.

We had both seen Michael Parkinson's television show on the same subject and, as journalists, agreed that it was a topic ripe for exploitation.

From then on it became irresistible to categorise all men over 35 in MM terms: candidates, sufferers, or escapees.

As time went by, however, superficial judgements gave way to a realisation that the MM was nothing like so lightweight a concept or ludicrous a condition as it had first seemed.

During the course of my research many men said it was a matter of serious concern to them, some openly admitting they felt they were losing their sanity and contemplating suicide — all because of the *'male'* *menopause*.

Anthea Linacre

Foreword

Anthea Linacre, one of the co-authors of this book, I have long acknowledged as a friend and respected as the only journalist I know who has complete professional integrity. Maybe this is because most of the journalists who approach me from time to time in my capacity as a sex-behaviour therapist (which entails being a psychologist) represent sensational newspapers who want smut. When I don't give it to them, because I can't — and if I could I wouldn't -- they are apt to make it up. Anthea has never done this; she has never reported anything I have told her "off the record", and has never misreported anything I have told her she may report. This makes her my favourite journalist.

So when recently, in a letter about something quite different, she threw in the statement: "I'm contemplating doing a book on the *'Male' Menopause* in collaboration with a man called Derek Bowskill", I had no compunction in writing back: "If you do this book I promise you I will tear it to shreds. There is no such thing as a male menopause in the sense of the female menopause. Men can be reproductive till the end of their days, and I get furious with people, especially GPs, who ought to know better, who put it about that men can be menopausal, since they are merely providing what I term "sex-lazy" men with an excuse for being just that".

However, I had forgotten that I had Anthea to reckon with. Yet I was not surprised when, a short time later, I had another letter sweetly asking me to do her and Derek the honour of writing an introduction to their book, thereby, I suspect she thought, drawing my claws. As I am not of a churlish nature I couldn't refuse, but I did reserve my stance. So here goes.

During the past forty years and more there has passed through my consulting-room a procession of women of all ages who have come to complain that their partners have lost all interest in sex. It is not that they are necessarily impotent, though impotence does feature quite extensively; it's just that when the partner indicates that she is sexually receptive, she is brushed aside with the classic excuse so often attributed to women, "Not tonight, dear, I'm too tired". Or the men themselves present, but unwillingly, and only because they hope that she is going to say, "Poor chap! Of course you mustn't have sex, you are tired, and this is a kind of tiredness for which there is no antidote".

Most of the men are in a state of nervous tension, and may feel disinclined for sexual activity as a result, though sexual activity, especially to climax, would be the best cure for their tensions. These tensions may produce irritability, too, and if they have a fluctuating blood pressure, they will periodically experience hot flushes.

These alleged menopausal manifestations are likely to occur at any age. Only a few months ago I had a patient of 23 who exhibited all these symptoms, and since he was married his lack of interest in sexual activity worried not only his wife, but himself. Yet the solution was in his own and his wife's hands. He wasn't impotent, and if he had *forced* himself into sexual activity, or let his wife produce all the action, the release from tension (the cause of his situation) would have removed all the symptoms. However, my "sex-lazy" man usually falls into the 45 — 55 age-group.

I agree entirely with Dr Michael Bott who, on page 148, maintains that what is commonly known as the male "menopause" is almost totally psychological in origin. Very very few cases have organic causes; for example, the lowering of the hormone level, which also allegedly affects the libido — the sex-drive or sex-urge — and produces impotence. In the half-dozen or so cases which I have decided should be referred for hormone replacement therapy after tests (which are still not easy to come by in Britain) there was an initial positive reaction which, in all six cases wore off after a month or two, still leaving me with the conviction that, honestly, the whole thing is "in the mind".

Three or four years ago I carried out some research into the nature of the sex-drive (libido) and with the help of nearly 400 couples I was led to the conclusion that the sex-drive relies only to a very small extent on sexual chemistry, and to a very large extent on the voluntary desire for sexual activity. The more sexually imaginative a couple are, the more frequently they want to, and do, make love. (High-libido people in the chemical sense are also the most sexually imaginative.)

From this I deduce — and I think I have proved — that where men complain of being "menopausal", they have lost the zest for sex, for one reason or another, *the least likely of which is chemical.*

Masters' and Johnson's findings have only confirmed my own observations made some years ago, that the earlier in life one is sexually active, and frequently, the later in life one remains so. This applies speaking comparatively, to low- average- and high-libido people alike, though high-libido people are usually so completely uninhibited, have such highly developed sexual imaginations, as I have just observed, and extract such intense enjoyment out of every facet of sex that they appear to have the edge on the others.

Those who are not acquainted in the practical sense with the psychology of sexual functioning do not appreciate the tremendous influence the mind has over the body's capacity to respond sexually. More than 90 per cent of all cases of premature or too rapid ejaculation, of failure to obtain and/or sustain an erection in a shared-sex experience, of loss of libido, of retarded ejaculation, of anaesthetic orgasm — all have psychological origins. This is also true, I am convinced from personal clinical experience, of the symptoms displayed by what I call the "sex-lazy" man.

I have suggested that the cause of "sex-laziness" is tension of one kind or another. A great many of my 45 to 55 "sex-lazy" men are either self-employed or executives in large concerns — industrial or what have you. The two categories come under great stress in their middle years and for one specific reason.

Roundabout 45 a man suddenly wakes up to the fact that in fifteen, or at the most twenty, years' time he is going to have to retire. For the self-employed this means that if he is going to have a reasonably comfortable retirement he must acquire capital which, when invested, will bring him an income which will cushion his old age. He, therefore, throws himself into his business, devoting most, if not all of his energy to making as much profit as he can.

The executive, of whatever rank, is on a pensionable basis. Most pension schemes are related to the last two or three years' salary earned before retirement. That is to say, the larger the salary in these final working years, the larger will be his pension. The executive, having suddenly realised this, goes into top gear to get himself as high up the salary ladder as he can before he is due to retire in two or three years' time.

The self-employed and the executive have one thing in common. Under the misapprehension that sex saps physical and mental energy — a leftover from the myth that the activity required to obtain an orgasm is weakening — and because they have decided to throw the whole of their energy resources into their work, they conclude that if they dissipate some of their energy in sex, they will be using up precious supplies of energy which, they believe, they could use to more advantage in their business operations. Within a short time of "giving up" sex, they find they couldn't perform even if they wanted to, because the sexual system needs to be kept in good tone in order to function at all.

The first thing they do, therefore, is to drop out of sex.

Since sex is so closely, but quite wrongly, associated in the minds of a great many men with tiredness, the tiredness which they experience after devoting all their mental and physical energies to their work, automatically, by a kind of mental *volte face* actually produces an aversion from sex. Often this aversion is an unconscious reaction, the man thus affected being the first to complain to his doctor that he has lost his libido and/or his ability to function sexually. When this happens, it adds to the tensions which the rat-race of his work induce, and makes his sexual situation worse.

Under such stress, it is no wonder that some men exhibit such symptoms as palpitations, irritability, lack of enthusiasm for anything but work, moodiness, hot flushes and so on. Nor is it only the self-employed and the executive grades who are thus afflicted these days. For the last few years I have had an increasing number of men in all categories of jobs coming to me with exactly the same problems, for which the employment situation is responsible. To be declared redundant at 50, whether you're working on the factory floor, driving the dust-cart or controlling the queues outside a cinema, is just as threatening and pressurising as those tensions which grip the self-employed and the executive.

Then there are other categories under which "menopausal" symptoms originate. Linacre and Bowskill have recounted the cases of two very well-known figures who, to their great credit, have described their experiences in extensive detail and allowed them to be published. One is Colin Wilson, who became world-famous overnight with his book *The Outsider* while he was still too young to cope with the burden which *sudden* fame imposes; and the other is the artist John Bratby R.A.

Neither case surprises me. I do not say this from professional pride, but from a fairly extensive professional experience of "all sorts and conditions of men".

Wilson is an highly intelligent and intellectual man. His "Outsider" was almost universally described as brilliant. (I was in a very small minority who found flaws in his thesis, only to be condemned by the so-called *cognoscenti* as jealous, nose-picking and even down-right ignorant.) Then, as he says, for some time afterwards he found himself in the wilderness. Compared with his first book, his second was "unsatisfactory", and his subsequent work was subjected to even more denigratory criticism.

As a writer of military and naval history, as well as a practising psychologist, I know precisely what the extensive anti-Wilson lobby meant to his morale as a writer and as a man. His reactions to it were exactly what I would have expected.

Let's admit it, Colin — as Dr Johnson proclaimed, "No one but a fool writes except for money". Dr J meant, I'm sure, real writers, not dilettantes. When you were, as you put it, "in the wilderness", not only your professional pride was hurt, but your next meal was in jeopardy. And no one — *pace* the poet starving in the garret (visions of Thomas Chatterton) — can write on an empty belly. (Thank god, publishers have recognised this and are prepared to sustain one's body during gestation of a "likely lad" by offering "advances" — non-sexual but financial — thereby hoping to stimulate one's soul.) It was no wonder, therefore, that when you were so viciously attacked for so long, you should think that the world had come to an end; and no wonder that you exhibited the symptoms you have so vividly described. BUT THEY WERE NOT MENOPAUSAL!

Bratby is in complete contrast with Wilson. Many artists of great talent at least appear to be extroverts, uninhibited, cocking a snook at convention. My experience is that this is usually a self-deluding pose.

According to the rules for artists of talent, sexual activity should have been taken in its stride by Bratby. Yet he came a cropper over a psychologically induced sexual situation — the very common or garden cause of middle-aged, non-imaginative sex; viz. he was no longer sexually satisfied by a contemporary wife, so to prove his essential manhood, took up with a partner very much younger than himself.

This is a sexually banal situation, but when it is indulged in by a man of such alleged artistic talent as Bratby, it becomes significant. Even more significant are his reactions to his situation.

He, like Wilson, felt that he was threatened, so he retreated into the haven of "menopausal" response.

For this is what "male menopausal" reaction is — a refuge from the ugliness of reality.

I am as dead against the concept of the male menopause as ever I was, but —

The authors of this book have, in my opinion, produced quite a brilliant piece of work. They have researched the subject in depth and they have recorded the results of their researches with considerable sharpness and utter integrity. I have referred in these few introductory remarks to only a small proportion of their findings.

I was afraid that a book called *The 'Male' Menopause* would encourage my "sex-lazy" men to be even more sex-lazy. I feel, however, that I can recommend it to my anathema-men, with the near-certainty that by reading it they will realise how stupid they are and will be prompted to jolt themselves out of their truly phoney non-sexual experience.

For no man, I am sure, will want to be classed with the cases so ably described in this book.

Robert Chartham, Malta

1 Is It All A Myth ?

I'm 45 — and what have I done with my life?
What have I to look forward to but a slow stroll to death?

a self-styled victim

Last year, half my patients were middle-aged men — all anxious and inadequate. Many of them volunteered what was wrong with them. They would say, 'I've got the male menopause'

a psycho-therapist

Over the months, as word got round that we were working on the 'male' menopause, we found ourselves button-holed — even cornered — by the many people who wanted to talk about this controversial subject.

There was, predictably, an enormous amount of jesting from men:

"Don't look further — I've got it!" "I've already had it!" "I'm 28, so when can I expect to get it?"

Women were equally responsive and very opinionated. Wives, daughters and mothers were all convinced it existed . . . and, what is more, knew several men who had it. One girl in her early twenties tackled us at a party:

Recently my father has been very irritable and depressed — with dizzy spells and hot flushes. My mother didn't dare tell him what she thought, so got him to our doctor on a pretext. The GP said, 'You've got the male menopause,' but didn't give him a thing for it. We don't want him living in a fool's paradise if he needs treatment. What should we do?

Occasionally, though, we were sought out by men who wanted to talk seriously about what they considered to be a really bad experience. One would describe his terrible despondency. Another would outline his frantic attempts to recapture his fast-disappearing youth. One or two men spoke graphically of both things happening together:

All the outward show is there; the vitality, the vigour . . . the envied essence of youth, if you like. But inside, it's all meaningless . . . drab and hollow.

Opinions were plentiful, but definitions and explanations were pretty thin on the ground. We were however inundated with descriptions. . . and always of two markedly contrasting types: the men who seemed to be rebelling by chasing youth, bright lights and girls: and those who seemed to be giving in by becoming withdrawn, lethargic, hypochondriacal. . . and impotent, in every sense of the word.

So let us look at these two types, turning first to the more obvious case; that of the man who tries to find refuge in a youthful persona entirely inappropriate to his age.

A signal symptom here is the low-level hair parting adopted to disguise the balding head. The weird placing of hair — at once eye-catching and self-defeating — is, actually and symbolically, typical of the 'Male' Menopause condition since it does nothing but accentuate what it is supposed to conceal.

Sometimes the man will go to the inordinate lengths and expense of a hair transplant or a toupee. But whether natural or false, his hair will seldom be left for long without attention from a furtive comb.

He may sport a hat (perhaps at a rakish angle with a mini peacock's feather) purchased after the style of his youth. Alternatively, he may become a dedicated follower of trends — frequenting young men's outfitters for over-tight suits, loud ties and lurid shirts. (A case history of this type can be found on p. 71) To give himself the added 'lift' he no longer gets from life, he may turn gratefully to platform soles and built-up heels. But he is no classical Greek actor in an elaborate, brilliantly-coloured costume; behind a dramatic mask with an amplifier built into the mouthpiece, and perched on splendid boots with soles several inches thick. He comes not from *Oedipus Tyrannus* but from *The Emperor's New Clothes* — and just like that sadly deluded fellow, he relies too much on external validation for his esteem.

To bolster his ego he turns to drink — and takes too much, too often. So, primed with alcohol and strait-jacketed in his trendy gear, he is reduced to shouting at the world, "I am here! Listen to me. Please pay me some attention!" and there can be little doubt that he has 'become as sounding brass, or a tinkling cymbal'.

Indeed, 'sounding brass' is an apt description of how he presents himself to women. There is all the noisy effrontery and the total absence of substance. His approaches — always to the youngest and most attractive women — are no more than acts of aggression in a lecherous mode; and in this, the menopausal victim is like the penis-exhibiting inadequates that are found in alleys and parks — except he operates from under cover. His tactic is to exploit the office party; to blow his squeaker in the face of an adolescent typist; to mingle in the crush at the bar to press his elbow into a young and liberated breast; and to join the dancing just to approximate his buttocks to those of any young thing who is careless enough to stand in line of his weaving fire. In mixed company, he will channel his proclivities for touching up into bottom smacking and pinching — a favourite form of expression since it is usually sanctioned by society in the name of bonhomie and exuberance.

Some men are driven further and will abuse the trust of a colleague's pubertal daughter and subject her not only to the smacking and pinching routine but also to tickling and cuddling. Here, he counts on the role of respectable-friend-of-father to protect him from exposure as he enjoys the flesh that symbolises for him what he has lost . . . and may never regain. His pathetic pretence of virile bravura is only a cover for the despair that stems from a feeling of inadequacy and impotence — and a suspicion that he is redundant, as a person and a man.

The second type is far removed from the ageing raver we have just looked at. A psychologist at one of London's largest teaching hospitals described the syndrome well:

I'm sure my girl friend's father is going through it. He shows every sign. Every week-end we see them we have to talk, talk, talk. He's become a hypochondriac overnight — and a real health-food freak as well. He's that depressed and disenchanted that it's impossible to spend either an enjoyable or a rational evening with him. He thinks there's nothing left in life any more . . . and in fact he's really got it made! But he sends out really bad vib's — and not only that . . . he'll spell it all out at length; loud and clear if you once give him the chance. It's pathetic and frightening at the same time — but it also makes you bloody angry. You see, there's nothing you can do to please him. Everything and everybody has suddenly gone wrong. It's as if all the lights have gone out and he's lost his way in the dark.

This second type, hypochondriac or not, attempts no disguise or subterfuge, but since his depressions — like those of all depressives — can rarely be relieved by another person, neither a listening ear nor a supporting shoulder will do any good. Far too often he will be suspicious and hyper-sensitive; critical and sceptical or everything. Anxious about his career and saddened by what he sees as all his lost chances (many of which were never real chances in the first place) he will be convinced of the futility of all things (including talking about his problems: "It's no good talking to anybody. I know that, I've tried it and it does no good. But I still can't help it. I've got to talk to somebody.") and totally overcome by gloom.

Whether the man belongs to the first or the second type makes little difference to people's attitudes. He may be ridiculed by those who don't understand and pitied by those who do, but for certain he will not be envied. There is a good chance that he will be patronised by all and sundry — including his family and friends. Indeed, perhaps *especially* by his family, since that may be the only way they can protect themselves from his hurtful onslaughts and embarrassing behaviour. Frequently the 'male' menopause sufferer will make demands upon their time, energy and psychological resources that cannot be met; his emotional requirements are such that his family can never win.

Generally speaking, the menopausal male walks a lonely road. He is too proud to accept informed sympathy — wanting only the superficial support of flattery. He is too ashamed to show his real feelings — and often siphons them off by appearing over anxious about his physical health, or exaggerating his emotional state until it can only be treated as a matter of jest. He is too anxious to feel good in his skin and too insecure to look himself in the face in case his identity should flee away and disappear as does a mirage to a man dying of thirst. He is often too afraid to confess anything of what he really thinks and feels to his best friends — if they are still talking to him — and too inadequate to dare approach either his wife or his GP with what he not infrequently knows to be his real problem. He feels a fraud, a failure and a premature candidate for the scrap heap.

> Thou hast nor youth nor age,
> But as it were, an after-dinner's sleep,
> Dreaming on both.

The 'male' menopause may be a dreamy sleep for some, but for others it is a terrible nightmare; harbinger of the autumn of an unlived life . . . the great disposer. And that is how it most often appears to the victims, their friends and relatives. But what about the professional clinicians; what do they think? Does the 'male' menopause really exist? Is it real or apparent? Are there hormonal changes? Does a man's body go through cyclical stages similar to a woman's? Is it psychological or organic . . . or both? Is it, perhaps, no more than the melancholia described by Hippocrates, the Greek 'Father of Medicine', nearly two thousand years ago? Or is it a 20th Century phenomenon; a malaise of the spirit . . . a stigmata of the psyche?

Most male doctors considered secondary impotence the most important factor in a possible 'male' menopause and, for many of them, hormone ratios provided the key.

Most female doctors considered the psychological aspects to be the most important and for them the most significant features were (a) the effect of the female menopause on the sexual partner; (b) our culture that creates mirror-symptoms in men generally; and (c) both elements working together.

Psychiatrists generally found the answer in either the man's early background or his present environment, but were not averse to acknowledging the importance of the female doctors' attitudes. Over all, their response to a possible hormone imbalance was that there was insufficient information — but even if it were proven, they would continue with their usual method of therapy.

Although the facts about organic changes are still in short supply and their significance a matter of debate (if not controversy), it seems sensible to consider the views of those specialists who claim there is a meaningful period of change for some men in mid-life that may be due to the direct effect of hormonal imbalance although, and they are the first to stress this, it occurs in only a very small fraction of men.

Our first medical opinion is from Dennis Friedman, a psychiatrist responsible for the psycho-sexual dysfunction clinic at St. Bartholemew's Hospital, London. His views on the 'male' menopause were expressed briefly in the *General Practitioner* in an article on *Impotence and desensitisation.*

'Male Menopause'
As a psychological entity this does not exist, although men in middle age are just as prone as women to depression, which may lead to sexual apathy. There are a number of men however, between the ages of 45 and 55, who report a sudden reduction in sexual activity associated with mild testicular atrophy. This represents the true male menopause, is organic in origin and is accompanied by loss of libido, irritability, hot flushes, loss of recent memory and impotence.

Here, Dr Friedman discusses the 'male' menopause from psychological and organic view-points.

The 'male' menopause is an organic disorder — not a psychological problem. It has its psychological features, of course: impotence, irritability, depression and apathy — even hot flushes. The same sort of symptoms that occur in women in fact, and it can be treated in the same way as one treats women — by hormone replacement therapy. It is important to note however that it is only 1-2% of men who suffer in this way. There are only very few men who have this abrupt change in middle life — which is one of the reasons perhaps why the male menopause is generally regarded within the medical profession as a non-starter. Many men who are depressed and also suffer from impotence associated with the depression are given drugs which help the depression but make the impotence worse. Recent research has shown that many of the drugs used in psychiatry have a direct effect upon the production of sex hormones — so these factors must be borne in mind. These men have psychogenic impotence in the first place and suffer from the drugs in the second and do not come into the category of the 'male' menopause proper. Those who do show a radical improvement when they are given male sex hormones by injection. They get better: they feel more wide awake and alert; their apathy disappears — and this includes their sexual apathy; and their irritability and depression also go. But it must be stressed that not every case of impotence should be treated with injections of male hormone. When this happens, quite a number do get better — but most of them don't. The reason being that there was probably no indication that the hormone was needed — and this is only shown when the levels in the blood are tested.

To give the patient hormone replacement therapy when he is already producing enough by himself does tend to damp down his own production because the hormone is being produced outside the body. His sex glands will slow down and it may take some little time before they function normally again — so it is not totally harmless. It is important therefore that any diagnosis should be confirmed by the finding of a low level of male sex hormone in the blood. Too seldom is this test done and perhaps the reason is that it is a difficult, complicated and expensive test that takes a long time for the technicians involved. But it is an important step in checking on whether the impotence is psychogenic or organic. One needs to know about the sex hormone level, and also to establish that there is nothing wrong with the mechanism, the nerve supply or the blood supply to the genitalia. If the patient says he can't get an erection under any circumstances — with his partner or anybody else, through fantasy, girlie books or even the morning erection and dreams — then one should begin to consider whether it is likely to be organic. And this means looking at all kinds of factors including the 'male' menopause — and under those circumstances it would be quite reasonable to undertake an endocrine profile.

I have found no evidence of a placebo effect with hormone treatment. All males who have become impotent — be it psychogenic or organic — are anxious and they attribute the problem to all sorts of things like increasing age, or an inability to live up to their sexual expectations, or a fear of inadequacy or failure. Once anxiety is introduced into the situation the problem becomes much worse. Any activity is impaired by anxiety — and once you've learned anxiety in the coital situation it's very difficult to unlearn it. The chances of a placebo response are therefore most unlikely.

However, the 'male' menopause is the least common form of male impotence. It is a definite, clinical entity relating to gonadal insufficiency in males between 45 and 55 who have small, shrunken testicles and who are producing insufficient male hormone. The term should not be used for all those men who at the age of 45 or so become involved in sexual relationships outside their marriage. That is a psychological problem that has to be called something else.

I really dispute that there is a special problem that happens to people in their 40's and 50's. I have come across no evidence for a separate entity that should be prepared for or can be treated. For that matter I'm not even sure that the phrase 'mid life crisis' is helpful. I'm not sure what it means anyway. Life is full of crises and whether you are going to be adversely affected by any of them depends entirely upon the personality of the individual. Crises will happen in the right circumstances at any age. If a patient comes to me and says he sees no reason for living because his sex life has come to an end or he couldn't see what it was all about any more, I do not see it as potentially the 'male' menopause. What may have happened is that he is a man who needs reassurance and requires admiration; who is not at all confident about himself and needs all kinds of cues — including sexual cues — to stimulate a response in others. And he will have arrived at a time of life when he discovers that he has got as far as he's going to get and he may become disappointed and jealous. This may lead him into being more competitive on the one hand yet feeling more and more threatened on the other by those he perceives as being more successful than he is. All sorts of anxieties may surface at this time — but they will always have been there — and he will show himself to be a person without sufficient internal resources to recognise that it may be time to stop trying to climb; to realise that he can depend upon his own self and not require outside stimulation. The chances are that he will not be able to continue being contented because he had a basic feeling of discontentment as a baby that was reinforced regularly through childhood.

Needing too many external factors in order to be able to get on with things and life; being dependant, wanting lots of attention and reassurance; thinking that he must produce favours with the people in power because he needs the admiration, and worrying that he will not always be able to produce them . . . all these are factors likely to cause breakdowns in mental health. These are the people who will require help.

In almost every case it is necessary to involve the man and his partner in marital counselling and the best results are obtained when both of them are strongly motivated towards getting the whole thing better. Usually there is much more than the presented impotence or the assumed 'male' menopause. For example, there is the secondary erective impotence which comes into the menopausal category and the man may state "Well; everything was fine until recently. I'm now 45 and when we came home from our summer holiday . . . suddenly it wouldn't work any more." Now that has quite clearly something to do with the marital unit. There may be many reasons but something in the marriage has provoked that particular symptom. One has to ask, "Is there some hostility? What has prompted the hostility?"

Another example: a male patient, 43, married for twelve years found he was unable to achieve erection or, if he did, was unable to maintain it. On taking the history I established that throughout the marriage the wife had been very inhibited and shy sexually. They had never had intercourse with the lights on — it had always been under the sheets, etc. And always after intercourse she had post coital cystitis. This meant that they couldn't have intercourse very often — and if they did she was ill the following day and for a week afterwards and had to be treated with antibiotics. On average therefore they were having intercourse once a fortnight. He thought their performances were OK, although he said, "In all the marriage, sex hasn't been all that good." Then the wife became better and when she found that she was no longer going to become ill she became far more interested in sex and actually started initiating and appearing demanding. The husband felt he was not going to be able to live up to her expectations: he was a man who was fine once a fortnight, but three times a week brought out his anxieties. This sort of case has nothing to do with the 'male' menopause — although a lot of wives may label it that way. It is merely an example of the fear of failure and the circular thinking that goes with it.

A further example of the same kind of self-defeating process is when husband and wife go to 'swinging' parties and the husband finds that he is unable to obtain erection with his partner while his wife is having intercourse with someone else. This may be a reflection of a history of always being left out of things in early family life. When he was growing up, everybody loved everybody else except him and there was, therefore, jealousy if mummy was upstairs having a good sexual relationship with whoever it might be . . . *and not loving him* . . . and this provoked hostility, and prevented him from feeling loving. And the same feeling occurred at the party: he was going to be left out; everybody else was going to be happy; and there was no changing his belief that it would always be like that. There are many reasons but some people are inadequate in the first place otherwise they wouldn't need to go and check their sexuality with multiple puppet shows.

In so many cases it is a matter of inadequacy — personal inadequacy — learned years back . . . and nothing whatsoever to do with the 'male' menopause proper.

Dennis Friedman took no exception to the phrase 'male' menopause, but there were many doctors who did. One who was particularly critical was Dr David Delvin, Medical Editor of *The General Practitioner* and author of *The Book of Love*.

It is very important to establish at the outset that there is no such thing as the 'male' menopause. Having made that clear, it is also important to recognise that patients themselves use the phrase. They do come along and say, "I've got the 'male' menopause," or, "My husband has got the 'male' menopause," and by that they mean one of two things — two clinical pictures which may merge into each other.

The first one is impotence. This may simply mean that the man thinks he has a hormone deficiency in the same way as his wife. She has developed the hot flushes and he has developed impotence.

The second picture is one of depression, anxiety and worry, dissatisfaction with himself, his wife, his job — or whatever.

There may of course be a combination of the two pictures in so far as the man who is fed up and depressed may well be impotent. It is hard to tell which is the commoner since it depends to a great extent on *where* you are when they present. If you are in a Family Planning Clinic the common pattern will be one of the wife complaining about the husband's impotence or, sometimes nowadays, the husband making a brave effort and coming in himself. If you are working in general practice it will be more common to see chaps who are feeling rotten and generally under the weather. Some of them may even be getting hot flushes — the same sort of symptoms as their wife.

I have come across a number of men with these symptoms, but it's not surprising when you examine it. Hot flushes come under the control of the emotions largely. People blush and go red with anger so it's not unlikely that the man will associate the hot flushes with the 'male' menopause. If he feels he's having the menopause, then he may start having the hot flushes. It's similar to those men who start having labour pains in sympathy with their wives — a straightforward example of couvade.

One can attempt to treat the hot flushes with hormones but very often they will go away by themselves — simply and without fuss. But it is important to remember there is no such thing as the male menopause when talking about hormones otherwise one gets the wrong picture. If you draw a graph of the fall off in male hormone production over the years it is not the same as with female production, which tends to fall off fairly sharply at about the time of the menopause. This will be around 48-49 depending upon the individual and it is this *sudden* fall off which creates some of the symptoms because the action of the pituitary gland is unopposed by the ovarian hormones for the first time. This causes the hot flushes and the night sweats.

In men, there is no sudden fall off in hormone production. It is incredibly gradual — far, far more gradual than most people imagine. The slight decline begins around age 40 and continues gradually for twenty, twenty-five, thirty years or so. There is no sudden crisis as there is in the female. However, there is no doubt that impotence is far more common in older men. 83% of sufferers from secondary impotence are over 40 and 75% are over 50. But it is complete nonsense to think that impotence is an inevitable consequence of ageing. There are plenty of men of 70 or 80 who are totally potent, so if a chap becomes impotent at 48 or whatever and says it is the male menopause — it isn't. It is almost always psychological. There are one or two physical causes — far less than people think — and they include diabetes, and blood pressure drugs. But, by and large, the impotence that comes on quite a few men in middle age is not the 'male' menopause. It is based upon a psychological origin and can very often be helped by straightening out their hang-ups. They should go with their wives to a suitable therapist and start talking out their difficulties. On the whole they fall into fairly well known categories.

Alcohol and obesity certainly play an important part. The phrase "Brewers' Droop" is famous for obvious reasons. But whether obesity plays a psychological or physical part is hard to say — probably both.

Perhaps the foremost important factor is overwork. Businessmen and self-employed chaps who are working their guts out till all hours just get too tired to perform. Business worries build up anxieties and many men become deeply concerned about being made redundant.

Then there is the factor of monotony. There is no doubt that this plays a part in generating a lack of interest in sex in both men and women. Difficult relationships between spouses make for problems in this area. If things aren't going too well then very often this leads to impotence. And if the wife has sexual problems on her own account this will be an influential factor — particularly if the wife has the very common condition of vaginismus so that her sexual muscles tighten up whenever any approach is made. It is quite remarkable how many women who have vaginismus are married to men with secondary impotence, be it partial or total.

Another factor may be that the woman has lost her attractiveness. It may sound harsh to say this, but if the wife has let herself go to seed — perhaps through no fault of her own — it may well produce impotence in the husband.

Then there is the fear of performance itself. This is very much part of the male machismo thing that men are supposed to perform well. If a man is frightened, it is difficult for him to get an erection. The more frightened he is, the more difficult it will be. Fear is the great enemy of erection.

As with all sexual hang-ups, there is always the question of the repressions that the man got during his childhood. Perhaps he was brought up to feel that it was all a bit nasty. These feelings may lie dormant in the back of his mind for thirty years and finally express themselves when he is 45 so that he thinks — albeit unknowingly — that he should be past all this rather nasty and distasteful business. If, as a child, he was fed the idea that people in their middle age shouldn't really go in for that kind of thing and that it is only to do with the procreation of children, then when he approaches that age himself he will begin to think that enough is enough. The attitude isn't as common now as it used to be but it still comes up even in otherwise apparently mature and broad-minded people.

Another fact, although not a very common one, is that of latent homosexuality. Sometimes they go off sex with a woman because they yearn for a man before it's too late. But more usually, they retreat into no sexual performance at all because the desired alternative of homosexuality is totally unacceptable to them.

Those are the factors which influence the impotence side of the picture. The other side, which as I have said may be mixed in with it, concerns the feeling rotten syndrome with all its odd symptoms including the hot flushes. And here we have something that is jolly common and the reasons for it are the same as those that give women psychological symptoms on top of their physical menopausal symptoms. At a certain age, somewhere between 45 and 55, it is difficult for men to come to terms with the fact that they are not so young as they were. It may sound simple and obvious but a lot of people overlook that it is difficult for a man when he realises that he is slowing up; that he is no longer as fit or as tough as he was; and that his children are beginning to run faster than he can. He is also probably beginning to realise that he has not made as much of a success of life as he had hoped to. His dreams may not be coming true. He may even be facing redundancy. He sees and knows that he is not as attractive as he was. He may be paunchier and balder than he was and not so appealing to women. He may also notice that his wife is neither as attractive as she was nor as terribly interested in him — and she may be running into health problems of her own.

All these factors promote a clinical picture in which there is anxiety, depression, irritability and very often insomnia. So there is a tremendous temptation to go to the doctor and say, "Oh, it's the 'male' menopause." But when he has a check up, the chances are that nothing specific will be found and the doctor will reassure him that it will pass and, if necessary, give him an anti-depressant which will hopefully buck him up and help him to sleep better. Then he should throw off the troubles quite rapidly, especially if he has a good relationship with his wife and family and his job is reasonably fulfilling and secure. I wouldn't honestly say that it is terribly common for a man to go on for years in the bad state. Most men do come to terms with it after a few weeks or months. I would say that most men can pull themselves round and my experience is definitely that one sees far less men with psycho-neurotic symptoms in GP surgeries than women. Women tend to suffer much more with the psychological overlay of the true menopause. They find it really difficult to adjust and this is reflected by the very high female consumption of tranquillisers and anti-depressants.

The commonest time for this male condition to present is in late 40's and early 50's. It is not to be confused with the well recognised involutional melancholia or depression that is to be seen in men and women at about retiring age. That tends to be more of a straightforward depression while this thing is much more nebulous. It is true that if one were able to give it some kind of name one could say, "This is what you're going through but don't worry it won't last for long. Let's have a chat about it." Perhaps male middle age anxiety — but 'male' menopause is absolutely ludicrous and not helpful at all.

Before we conclude this introductory survey of opinions from those who are after all merely observers, perhaps we ought to include some comment from the victims themselves. It will help keep in perspective the dispassionate tone that has so far controlled our outlook. Here are a few quotes, mainly taken from the case histories and personal statements that appear later:

I reviewed what I felt about life, people, things — and above all, me. And I discovered that all I had had for some time was a sense of depression and dissatisfaction with life generally. A sense of kicking against the pricks. A sense of questioning one's virility — and one's sexual attractiveness.

John R. . . . . . .

This ancient medico said 'Well, it's what you have to expect. You are, after all, coming up for the meen-o-pause.' I just thought, Christ!

Roger D. . . . . . .

You're dead right men get the bloody menopause. Listen here: men demand the right to the fucking menopause! Look at me; I still like writing . . . but all I really think about is fucking and boozing . . . there's nothing else like it. But come the menopause it will all go. Come the menopause there will be nothing left. Come the menopause it will be 'PISS OFF'. That's what it will be. 'PISS OFF'. It's too true; men do get the bloody menopause . . . and what's more they bleed. I've been bleeding for two years now . . . too bloody true!

Geoff Nuttall, author of 'Bomb Culture.'

If you get through it, I think you have a good chance of going on and thriving. But when it strikes — in the 40's as it does — it strikes with a force that can provoke panic or paralysis.

Colin Wilson

The sort of traumas that are associated with the 'male' menopause can drive you mad. You may not appear to be mad, not outwardly, but they can drive you right out of your mind.

John Bratby

In the face of such comments as these and the revealing personal statements from men and their families that come later, it is difficult not to accept that *something happens*. We would suggest that it is equally difficult not to accept that what happens to men can be perceived by them as the *'male' menopause*. Although the experts may disagree about whether it happens or not and about what to call it, the terminology seems to speak for what men feel they experience. Friends, wives, doctors and agony columnists, as well as many others, tell of hundreds of men who define their problem as the 'male' menopause. It may be careless thinking or loose language. It may be a cliche of the media or a myth of the collective male consciousness. It may be men's rebellion against the supposed liberation of women or it may be women's way of putting men down. It may be inexact, inappropriate and faintly ludicrous. It may even appear vulgar or obscene to some of us – but it does work. It is illuminating. It does cast a telling meaning over what happens to many men in their middle 40's – and, most significantly and usefully, it does inform us all about what they *feel* is happening to them . . . weird overtones and all, since for many men, it is the overtones that play havoc with their lives. So, from here on, we shall not use quotation marks or italics when we refer to the male menopause, nor shall we prefix it with *quasi, so-called* or *sort of.* It will now stand on its own merits – complete with overtones, undertones, confusions, complexities and rushes of blood to the brain. In fact, we are suggesting that the phrase is meaningful in so far as it defines and describes a syndrome that is self-contradictory . . . and perhaps self-defeating. Perhaps, too, the use of the terminology is self-destructive for the individual who believes himself to be a victim and we are not insensible that the use of the phrase for the title of this book may add fuel to a fire that some would say is improperly burning – and should never have been lit in the first place. But it has been lit and it is burning with hot and high flames, and we therefore see it as our job to look more closely into them and not just to stand back with the patronising smile of superiority saying, "Of course, there is no fire. I don't know what all the fuss is about," nor to run away in panic shouting, "Fire, Fire".

In the past, and in many other cultures even today, a man could rely on age to bring him some respect. Even if he had gained little esteem during his early years and had done little to deserve or justify even the smallest bubble of reputation, he could rest assured that middle age would earn him some respite from stress and strain and he would reap the minimum reward of his society accepting that he would, "grow wiser and better as my strength wears away".

Times have changed — and they did so dramatically with the socio-cultural explosion of the 50's in Britain. Since those brilliant years, age and experience have stood for nothing in our collective view of what is worth having and doing. To be middle-aged is almost worse than being old. The middle years symbolise middle of the road achievement and middle class values — qualities no longer held at a premium. Ever since the 50's it has been youth and vitality to which we have paid homage. Experiment and even anarchy seem to command more attention and offer greater rewards than any of the traditional attainments and accomplishments of middle age. What were once the virtues and worthwhile tributes and attributes of middle age no longer stand as consolations for the fear or grief of a possibly waning virility; nor can they in a society that is besotted by the constant titillations of our sex-obsessed media. There is little wonder that so many people who have talked to us have equated the male menopause with secondary impotence when there are so many false models of sexuality paraded before us. Men are presented as handsome studs who can perform at the drop of a trouser and recover their vital strength again, and again, and again . . . and women are portrayed as near-automatic responders, ready to fling themselves about in frenzies of ecstasy akin to an attack of major epilepsy, and to continue so doing through their multi-orgasmic, hours-long session. Novels and films have much to answer for not because they offend by their frankness, but because they mislead with their 'thrusting' cliches of quasi-sexuality that are based upon plastic passion. Failure to live up to such models can have a disastrous effect upon men of any age (and women too, but generally they are too sensible to take much note of silly myths) but when the feeling of inadequacy in sexual relationships develops at the same time as an urge to self-questioning, it can be tragic.

It is ironic that it is no comfort to most men to know that their sexual powers were waning from their early 20's, and in some cases, before — so the actual decline, no matter how gradual, has been going on for years. However, it presents itself to them as a new feature because of the comparative effect. There are few men who have enjoyed as active or as experimental a sexual life as they would have wished. As Paul Rimmer points out on p.102, many men would like to have been Errol Flynn — and there are not many who do not regret that. To such men, it is likely that the first suggestion that they might fail when involved in love-making (as opposed to merely failing to have sufficient opportunities for what they think they might have liked) would prompt a bitter taste of resentment.

It does seem possible that the male menopause is a direct result of our present pre-occupation with the young as sources of wealth and leaders of fashion and culture. The gilded vessel with 'Youth on the prow, and

Pleasure at the helm' carries no message of comfort for those fearful men who, gripped by a sense of inadequacy, are struggling in a crisis of confidence and nearly ready to give up completely. Nor is the panorama of over-active youth anything but a threatening challenge to those who have decided to rebel against the encroachment of middle age by flaunting reality in a desperate attempt to 'go it alone' back to better days. Whether resigned or rebellious, our fixation on effervescent immaturity brings nothing but unhappiness to those men who feel that things are not what they should be, nor what they used to be . . . and nor, for that matter, are they.

> Youth like summer morn, age like winter weather;
> Youth like summer brave, age like winter bare.

. . . the comparison may not be difficult for an aged man to take. His process of change is complete and he is well on his way to accepting the, albeit ridiculous, parameters of the human condition, birth and death for what they are — the only absolutes. He may well be secure in his anticipation of death, and he may be able to approach it with equanimity — after all, winter is winter. But for the menopausal male there is no such security (and no man who suffers from the menopause is capable of accepting that the only security known to us comes from an understanding of the total insecurity of all things except death); he is trapped between his memories of spring and summer and his fears of a winter for which he feels woefully ill-equipped. For him, autumn is all: the pale sun casts long shadows before him and its rays have lost their ability to warm — they come from too far away; his evenings are damp; his future seems bleak or lost in a fog; and he has only a meagre harvest to contemplate — and that is already mainly reaped . . . and rotting.

All of us have our dreams and many of us set our hearts on certain goals. Some of us want our photographs taken in front of 10, Downing Street, but most of us are aware, even at an early age, that we won't set the world on fire . . . but we don't agree to settle for less than starting some kind of flame, somewhere. It may be playing for Leeds United (or Scunthorpe Reserves); it may be writing a best-selling novel (or a letter to The Times); or to sail round the world (or down the French canals). It is the discovery that our cherished dream will not come true that creates the Walter Mittys and the Billy Liars of this world . . . and the menopausal males.

It comes as a crisis of confidence; perhaps a final and extreme one when all our previous, precious confidence has been based not on what we actually were . . . but on what we might become. Now, Sartre was right when he suggested that it was what a man might become that was more important than what he was — but his growth depended upon him being something in the first place. If a man is no more than a collection of dream possibilities, when the last vestige of hope for realising these dreams disappears, the man disappears also. He does not suffer an identity crisis. He experiences for the first time in his life his total absence of personality. An identity crisis presupposes more than one persona, and any consequent tension stems from problems of choice — much less of a castrating experience than coming face to face with . . . no face, no persona, NO SELF.

Some of our authorities take this revelation so seriously that they suggest it is responsible for a number of successful suicide attempts by menopausal males. They do not claim that the menopause itself is responsible for the death wish, but that it is the catalyst that allows the man's early psychological history to catch up with him. He then over-responds to the stresses. Men who have had an early history of flaws or failures of confidence; men who felt inadequate, deprived or unloveable in childhood; and men whose internal reservoirs of self-esteem were never initially filled nor properly serviced later are likely to attract and become totally fouled up in the menopausal crisis. (This is a point that many of our contributors stress, particularly Sidney Wasserman — please see p. 44.)

Some men hold on to their dreams for much longer than one would think possible in the face of the harsh winds of reality, but some become resigned to a dreamless, aimless, normless existence very early on — almost in the first flush of adolescence. Some of them have little choice; their secondary school careers have been long journeys of discovery that bring them to the common destination of disenchantment. There are many young men (and women) who are told days in and out for the whole of their secondary education that they are without talent, hope or potential — and some of them believe it. So, if you have had your crisis of short-fall in adolescence there is no opportunity for you to come face to face with a bad reality. After such a rotten start, things can only get better.

Also, some authorities believe that the male menopause might be a man's second adolescence, so if his total development was arrested in his first there must be every chance that for him the menopausal kick-back will be precluded. "They who would be young when they are old must be old when they are young," is a well-known saying, and whichever way you look at its meaning, it is not a cheerful prospect.

Having touched upon education, perhaps we ought to see it through — and look at the reverse of the coin. For example, is it possible that the classic candidate is to be found in the ranks of teachers? "Those who can, do; while those who can't, teach," may be of particular relevance to menopausal victims. Certainly, it seems a sickness that feeds upon thwarted ambitions and frustrated drives, and those who man our educational system are among the most thwarted and frustrated in the world. All levels of education — primary, secondary and tertiary — are riddled with the living dead who try to compensate for their own ontological insecurity by exercising power over those without the wherewithal to fight back or even resist. The petty standards of self-validation through the eyes of society's prejudices and hypocrisies are to be found in many classrooms and lecture halls, while resentment, distrust and disillusion rule the day in staffrooms peopled by strait-jacketed bodies below faces obscured by masks.

Teachers are supposed to be holding up standards that are worth pursuing through a lifetime and most of them found long, long ago that their evaluations were false — but they are lacking in the courage to give up a pension and the kind of security and authority that being a pedagogue stands for. Their condition is exacerbated by their career structure, where the *good* teacher's only way of promotion lies in moving out of the classroom into a world of pseudo administration. In too many facets, therefore, is it a profession for seconds, and the menopausal victims are countless in the 'not quites' who know they will never become more than assistants. They are the lecturers who discover they are not going to make it as professor and the teachers who are never going to be Heads — or get a college appointment. (Assistant Managers who are not going to be promoted Manager, and Deputies who are not going to achieve a seat on the Board also qualify, but the ethos of their business organisations is not in itself menopausal — as it is in the teaching profession.)

However, the men are not entirely ciphers or they would not be candidates in the menopausal stakes. To qualify, a man does need a basic level of awareness and some powers of objectivity in assessing self-development, but the level must not exceed that above which a realisation of what should be done would dawn, otherwise he would be out of the condition. In brief, too little awareness and the man will never catch it; too much and he will quickly discover his own antidotes.

The farm-worker, the deep sea fisherman, the builder's labourer and all others who depend simply upon physical efficiency to bring in their bread are more than aware of the impact of middle age — especially those employed on piece work. But for them there is no menopausal tension, just the need — no doubt bitter and unwelcome, but clear and plain — to accept the fact that they are in time's hands and there is little they can, or could ever, do about it. It may be a time of sadness for lost powers, but their grief is a natural one for a normal process — and not tainted with recriminations and self-doubt.

In fact, some men seem to escape the menopausal syndrome altogether and they are the ones who measure their own success, achievement and growth by their own standards. They may also be successful in the eyes of the world, but the essence of their escape from the male menopause is to be found in their own esteem, their own values and their own self-images. Subjectivity is paramount here since many menopausal men have 'made it'; according to our society's standards they have created fulfilling lives and have assembled around themselves all the features that the good life has to offer: big houses expensive cars, attractive wives, pleasant offspring and a job with apparent power and no shortage of money. The truth of the situation is that these values reflecting a gross, acquisitive attitude, do not in the end add up to a life that meets man's better aspirations — and many of the men who achieved the top of that particular ladder find it empty and desolate. (James Hemming has a lot to say about this top-of-the-tree rat race on p.156.) It is the man's opinion of himself that will dictate whether or not he will suffer badly from the ravages of the menopause.

Let us look, then, at some men who feel they have avoided the male menopause. Colin Douglas, well known for his performance in *A Family At War,* is now 63. This is what his wife said. "I don't think Colin ever really suffered it. There was one time when he worried about whether he might be going to die — but I wouldn't call that menopausal. Perhaps one of the things that helped prevent it was marrying slightly later in life than average. He was 38. I was then 23 and I think that is another factor in warding it off: having a young wife. You see, when Colin was 45-50, I was 30-35, and I am sure that helped."

Another point of view, this time from a man himself, is expressed by Tony Britton. At the time we interviewed him, his performance as *The Nearly Man* had prompted many people to suggest that the character was menopausal. One of the ironies of our research was to discover that Tony Britton's portrait was being painted at that time by John Bratby whose own contribution so dramatically compares with that of his sitter. Here is Tony Britton's appraisal of the condition.

I'm very fortunate in that I still feel about 18; I still feel that I've got a lot to learn, and I still feel that there's plenty of time. I'm fortunate in that my drive, my energy and my wish for achievement haven't gone, and when you still have drive and energy you never really come to the end of the road. There is always somewhere else to go — some other road to take.

But I know that some middle aged men tend to feel quite sensitive about hair and teeth falling out, or going white and grey and they think, "I must dress young," and all that sort of thing — not to hold on to the faded remnants of youth so much as to hang on to middle age itself. Some of them start leaping into bed with secretaries. Well; a man always feels like that from puberty until the day he dies at 85 — so it's the desperation stage I don't really understand. I have great sympathy for it, but I don't understand it.

Everybody says the 'Nearly Man' was male menopausal — a man who has devoted twenty odd years of his life to an ambition he has failed to achieve. He is an intelligent man and aware that his failure is due entirely to his own weaknesses. So he compensates for that and a not so good marriage by having a girl-friend on the side. As *The Nearly Man* came to realise in the last episode, a man can reach middle age and review his life saying, "God Dammit; I've missed out." Well that's tough, of course, but he may have been responsible for an awful lot of it himself, and what he needs to say is what *The Nearly Man* said, "Well, that's it. I've made my mistakes and I've balled it all up so I might as well face the fact that I haven't got it and I may never get it now. Make the best of a bad job and just get on with it."

All this I can see, but for an intelligent guy to start ringing up the Samaritans in the middle of the night from that kind of depth of despair about failure and success and whatever I don't really understand. Maybe it will hit me when I'm 60. Maybe when I'm impotent one day I shall say, "Oh Dear God." — but I don't think so. I think I'll say, "I've got my family to love and care for. There's the garden, and I've got my books . . . and I might try to write." What I'm really saying is that the male situation is menopausal from puberty onwards. That's what I really think. We're dying from the moment we're born, and the pressures are on from adolescence. To a certain extent they're tougher then because you are ill-equipped and unaware. But the process of acceptance and adjustment goes on from puberty onwards.

For myself, there are still lots of things yet to be achieved. I'd absolutely adore to be known as an international actor. I'd like to make a lot more films; to work in America; and to do a play on Broadway. I hanker after directing and writing. I would have loved to have been an Oscar winner — but I must confess the older I get the less important it is to have these baubles on your mantlepiece. I no longer take them seriously. What is still serious is being as good as you can at the job and being recognised for that by the public and the people who employ you. As an actor you never stop learning so you've always got that. You can never stop and say, "I am now the complete, perfect actor." If you found yourself saying that you would give in straight away because there would be nowhere else to go . . . and anyway it's not true. You can never get it quite as good as you wanted it to be, never. So there's always that Golden Carrot dangled before the eyes.

I'm not dismissing all the propositions about the poor, unfortunate chaps who get this menopause. The fears are real fears and we all get them. They gradually happen one by one as you get into middle age and they may take a bit of accepting and adjusting to. You can see it all beginning to slip away. One day you look in the mirror and you see all the lines and wrinkles and you may throw up your hands in horror and say, "Oh Dear God; here it is . . . it's on the way". But life still goes on. One still carries on working and gradually you realise . . . that it is only you who takes an extreme view of what you see in the mirror. Other people accept you compeltely. They still give you work to do. You still go on being married . . . and you still go on doing those things you wanted to do in life; you still earn a living, you still go to parties; and you still find attractive young women coming to interview you for books!

There is also the eternal basic situation where for some reason or another, the older man is always an object of attraction to the younger woman. So there is that sort of comfort as well. And, of course, I am in a profession to which there is no end. Actors don't retire at 65. We're like old soldiers: we never die — we just fade away. And I suppose I am being a bit bloody selfish when I say I don't understand about men with menopausal problems. The truth is that I am a very lucky man; a favoured man. Most men of my age are not lucky enough to be doing a job that they still absolutely adore and which fulfils them completely.

Many of the self-confessed victims of the male menopause we met were homosexuals. A moving personal statement from one such man is to be found on p.110. It shows how deep the despair can be, and he suggests that homosexuals are hit harder than other men when they fall victim to the condition. We turned to Quentin Crisp, author of *How to Have a Life Style.* At 67, he was able to look back on a lifetime as an effeminate homosexual, and he painted another picture for us.

My problem has never been a legal one. I've never taken any notice of the law. No; my problem has been how to get on with the world while flouting its conventions. How to have my cake and eat it, and this, to a little extent, I have now done. Of course, it is nonsense to pretend that I have become a totally acceptable being. There are still thousands of households where I would not be welcome for the same old, boring reasons as before . . . but I am free now. I do have a wider horizon. And to a certain extent life is easier just because I am older. One of the pleasures of ageing is that towards the end of the run you can over-react appallingly and this is what I now do. All the terrors that I might eat with the wrong fork are past and I am now quite happy to ask, "Which fork do I eat with?" Openness makes it all easier. People build up to such a lot of untruths about themselves that they live in terror of what might transpire if it was found out that their mother was not the Duchess of Thing. These people have a great deal to lose, but right from the beginning I had nothing essential to lose. I was, of course, easily embarrassed whereas now it would take a helluva lot to embarrass me. Also, when you are young, you have a different attitude to death. Then, it is a kind of Keatsian experience: you long for it but don't actually think you'll be dead. You think you'll look down from your cloud and count the number of people at your funeral.

I remember I once said to a woman, "I really can't get used to the fact that I will ever die," and she replied, "Neither can I, but I practise like mad." And this is what you must do. Dying takes a lot of practice. But in the end you have to come to terms with it -- and I think that most people of my age are frankly waiting for death.

Someone once said about me, "What makes Quentin so sad is that it's all complete. There isn't any more." Well, I suppose that that is fair enough but I see it more as a cause for rejoicing. I mean, I would hate to have reached the age I have and think, "I once thought I would have a house on the Isle of Wight and now I think I will die and never have had it." I think that would be a terrible situation.

There are other traps for the middle-aged to fall into. There is the dream that everything would be fabulous if only the man could have an illicit liaison with a red-haired Chinese woman on a green bicycle on a Wednesday. But as she's not Chinese or it's Thursday or something, that wonderful situation never arises. What he really needs to settle for is that when you are 50 you can only get out of life what your character will stand — and you can only get out of sex what your nervous system will stand. By the time you are 25 you've had what you're going to get in the way of sexual experience. As Mr Huxley said, "Refinement of technique does not produce refinement of sensation."

Another trap is for the middle-aged boss to start rushing after his secretary. All he will do is make himself feel older, because his secretary will be nice to him because he is her boss — and nothing can make you feel older than that, surely? So any scrabbling around after proof that you are still sexually potent is a complete waste of time as I see it. If you are an effeminate homosexual, you recognise you're ageing much quicker. A man of 45 knows that the dear little thing in him cannot be seen, cannot even be recognised any longer. So you re-arrange your life. You no more consider yourself as a nymph pursued by satyrs, or any of that rubbish. You become free to regard all people as people and as men and women, because your primary interest in them has become for their character and their capacity for friendship. You no longer have this dream of yourself as a desirable sex object. You don't expect to be loved more than other people. The most you ask is not to be betrayed or scored off. That is the positive aspect.

There is also another side. There is the fact sexually, rather than having to face up to the fact that you are becoming impotent, you have to accept that your sex drive remains the same while you become less acceptable. I am now 67 and my sexual processes haven't changed at all. In my opinion they just don't change, they remain the same. If ageing is tragic in any way it is not in the waning of sexual desires but that they stay where they are and that you become a funny old queen if you're homosexual or a dirty old man if you're not. People will say of a man of 55 who is marrying a woman of 40, "Well, I suppose they want the companionship," which is a load of rubbish. What they want is the sex just like anybody else. Possibly less often, but what with all the concealment and all the boasting you never really know whether you are under or over-sexed — which does make homosexual relationships more interesting because you can at least compare yourself with someone whose sexual processes are vaguely similar to your own.

The question of comparisons and judgements is at the root of all these things whether they are to do with ageing or sex. There is the story of the three magistrates that shows the difference in attitudes that people can have. A man is brought before them for having an illicit relationship with a goat and the man's counsel says, "This man's wife has been in hospital for a month." The first magistrate says, "Why have they dragged the fair name of this woman into court?" The second says, "Well; this might be an extenuating circumstance." The third says, "Oh, why didn't anyone tell me? Give him another goat." So you see; it's all in the mind.

As far as I'm concerned there is no menopause for men. There is no crisis whatsoever unless you like to regard every day as a crisis. What I really long for is my appetites to pass so that one day I shall be totally free.

Quentin Crisp must stand alone on many counts, but on the grounds of failing sexuality he is definitely removed from the sufferers from the male menopause. As we have already mentioned, for many men their menopause is no more and no less than a synonym for impotence. A diminishing sex drive is distasteful to many men, as is the thought that they may be losing their sex appeal — especially if they have valued, perhaps exclusively and excessively, themselves only in their sexual roles. Many men worry quite unnecessarily that they are losing their sexual attractiveness; and many more worry equally unnecessarily when they discover that they have lost it. For both groups it is as if they had no identity as a person but only as a sex object — and this, of course, may reflect their attitude to women. They may never have got past the stage when they saw women only as 'birds of prey'.

When a potentially menopausal male finds that, for the first time in middle age, he can't make love — even though it may be because of too much to drink or a working day of fourteen exhausting hours — he is often horrified and terrified. In his youth he may have laughed it off if it were drink or shrugged it off if it were over-tiredness, but in his middle forties it can seem an immediate and doom-laden omen for the future.

A single sexual failure (because inability to achieve an erection, to sustain one or just to fail to ejaculate is usually seen as failure — and there lies a significant moral) may be sufficient to trigger off intimations of menopausal gloom, and other isolated, perhaps more dramatic, events may also do the same. The death of a friend of a similar age or perhaps a heart attack may precipitate the symptoms and convince the victim he is on the way out . . . and soon. It is, unhappily, a self-perpetuating condition that encourages the growth of a self-fulfilling prophecy; I think I have had it . . . ergo, I very shortly have. The screw turns and the spiralling process completely takes over.

Redundancy is another stark factor that may precipitate it all. Or, at a less severe level, the realisation of the short-fall of career or other life goals as mentioned earlier. Since men place such importance on their sexual and work roles perhaps these two factors must rate most highly among those that cause the beginnings of the menopausal syndrome. For many men, the future holds nothing more than retirement and death — because that is how they see it, and once they have given in to that kind of thinking, serious mental and emotional stress can follow straight away.

The fear of death comes to some men as a total experience and it is the loss of awareness that worries them most. They value themselves as thinking, feeling persons and the *passing by of self* brings them no pleasures of anticipation. Others, allowing physical vanity to rule their lives, see total death almost from the first wrinkle. By tradition, beautiful women are often hit brutally by the menopause, and, by the same token, vain men will suffer more from the early signs of physical decay. In fact, a lifetime of vanity may bring them disaster in, for them, a particularly cruel Nemesis of failing features.

Our menopausal victim, vainer or not than most, is in danger of confusing natural ageing and decay with sinister signs and omens. The aware man will be able to detect the difference, but others may not. (In fact, the testimony of Dr Hoche, on p.170 asserts that differentiation often eludes the experts). Gerard Manley Hopkins in *The Leaden Echo* takes a dramatic stand:

> Do what you may do, what, do what you may,
> And wisdom is early to despair:
> Be beginning; since, no, nothing can be done
> To keep at bay
> Age and age's evils, hoar hair,
> Ruck and wrinkle, drooping, dying, death's worst, winding sheets,
>   tombs and worms and tumbling to decay;
> So be beginning, be beginning to despair.
> O there's none; no no no there's none:
> Be beginning to despair, to despair,
> Despair, despair, despair, despair.

It would appear that youthful complexes may return at this menopausal second adolescence to haunt the man with a vengeance that he has not experienced since puberty. For example, a small man we talked with told us how inferior he felt because of his height and it was not until he was 26 and met a very small girl who fell in love with him that what he called his 'trouble' began to fall away.

I thought my trouble was dismissed to Limbo. But now twenty years later, I've got the menopause starting and all my old fears have come pouring back. I just yearn to be tall – all over again – so that women would find me more attractive. It's not that my wife doesn't love me or anything like that. She still thinks I'm a pretty good fellow. But it doesn't make any difference.

The aspect of how early complexes and deprivations, fears and anxieties may affect a menopausal man is something that our next contributor stressed. He is an external lecturer at the Universities of Bradford and Leeds and also undertakes in-service training courses with the Social Services Departments in Sussex, Berkshire, Reading and Wakefield. He says of himself, "I'm a bit of a peripatetic social worker. I keep saying that I have a motto, 'Have casebook – will travel' ". He is the author of a paper, "The middle-age separation crisis and ego-supportive casework treatment".

What triggers off the male menopause in many cases is a feeling of deprivation. "I got cheated. It's not what I really wanted." The man often thinks the problem is his marriage partner – she wasn't the right one. And then it grows into a resentment that his kids haven't turned out to be the fulfilling ones he hoped they would. And when the obsession begins to grow, it spreads rapidly until he says, "Dammit; there's only so much time if I'm really going to make it now – in work, leisure time and with women – I've got to make a killing before it's too late. Since we live in an age of permissiveness and since my wife isn't going to make it for me or with me and since everything tells us that we can obtain fulfilment if we grab for it, then I'm gonna grab. I'm gonna grab things and I'm gonna grab people and I'm really going to get what's coming to me."

What really happens with many men is that they are warding off an inner depression. They have an emptiness, a void and many men get obsessed with trying to fill it in. Some do it with young girls – but responding to the compulsion isn't very satisfying. The man may get a momentary reassurance but he is in fact trying to fill a bottomless pit so he must go on and on. And after one affaire or a one night stand he feels guilty and depressed so in order to ward that off he has to find somebody else. Before you know it he is on a spiral that is almost an addiction and he just can't stop. Part of the trouble is that today's society expects you to conform to this pattern. You're expected to keep your nice wife and family all sweet on the surface but to have your mistresses and whatever on the side. The working class man may handle it differently through drinking heavily with the boys and his wife may accept it, but she gets squeezed out in another way.

The real problem we must address ourselves to is how to help an individual who is trying to deal with a gnawing grief and depression that is related to a much earlier time in life. What the man is actually saying is, "My mother didn't love me enough." He is now at a point in life when he feels it is his last chance to get that love but he may not even be aware that he is still seeking some kind of maternal fulfilment. The deprivation may be real or imaginary, but if he perceives it as deprivation then it really is so for him, and he will remember that he was always overlooked or replaced and somehow, no matter what he did, he could never please her. Nothing was ever enough. And he often repeats that situation with his wife. He tries to handle it by giving her a second car and lots of clothes — but basically he still feels that he isn't really satisfying her because deep, deep down he feels unloveable. He compensates for this feeling of not being loveable by sort of grabbing and acting out. Of course, it doesn't work and some of the men literally have a total breakdown.

It's very painful to say, "I don't feel loved", or "I'm not loveable", and it takes a certain degree of maturity to be able to do that. And what happens in the male menopause is that instead of developing that level of maturity, there is a regression back to an earlier level. Sometimes the man can work through it with his wife. Sometimes he might say, "Well, look here, I'm not going to fill this void inside me so I've got to accept what I am and what I've got. What I have got is my wife and she's all I have so I'm going to settle for that." Now, the thing is that it is not a one-way street and the wife can exacerbate the situation for the husband if she doesn't read his signals correctly. She may be going through the same business, "My youth is going. I'm fading. I'm no longer attractive." She will be feeling useless, perhaps because of the end of her fertility and she may also be worried about the end of her sexual life — plus all the social myths about her own menopause. This will complicate her reaction to the husband at this time. She may withdraw into herself and he will read it as a withdrawal from him of her love. She may start putting the pressure on him with higher expectations and he will interpret this as, "She doesn't really care about me. All she wants me for is what I can give her in material things and she wants to exploit me." So the merry-go-round goes on. In many ways she will be struggling with feelings of depression and grief for her lost youth and fertility, and she may respond, "I've got to grab. I didn't get all I wanted and if I don't get it now before my attractiveness goes it will be too late."

When this kind of situation sets in, many men become impotent with their wives. They don't know that what they are really doing is expressing their feelings of tremendous rage associated with their mother from early days. They withold from their wives what they think they want, and often act it out grabbingly by trying to knock down as many women as they can. It looks like sexuality but in fact it is rage and aggression about women planted by his unfulfilling relationship with his mother. One mustn't dismiss the fact either that as the woman gets older, for some men she gets too close to the mother's age, as it were, and so it is almost like having intercourse with his own mother.

There is also the man's own ageing process and some men over-respond to this by driving themselves into an athletic heart. Others will become sad but philosophical. And yet others will produce a reaction formation like, "I'm not sad about it at all. It's what I've been waiting for: to be older, wiser and for my grey hair to give me dignity." The trouble is that, as a society, we don't bring any of this out into the open. It's like the elephant in the room that nobody talks about. It's just like death — a taboo subject. I suppose that things have improved a little in the last 10 years but we need to air it much more — to give people plenty of time for early preparation. We do a lot of educating of society about children and adolescents — but not about middle age and they need it the most because they are caught between the generations. They are often pulled apart by aged parents on the one side and the kids on the other. It can be a real dilemma.

Some men get out of it by changing jobs and getting off the affluent rat race. But for others, the changing of jobs — the rushing and flailing about — is merely another form of chasing girls. They get busy chasing jobs instead of looking into what is really wrong. Neither changing jobs, wives or conquering birds will do any good if you had heightened feelings of deprivation and lack of fulfilment in childhood which have been reinforced through the years. But what the man can do is to grieve his lost childhood in a way he never did before. Often, that will free his energy to get on with life and complete it. He has every right to grieve what he didn't get but our society doesn't sanction men grieving. Men aren't offered the channels to mourn, and they pay a very great price in this culture for the inability to say "Look here, I want to be loved. I feel unloved and I want to cry because I'm not loved." If a man can go through this grieving with his wife, the help can be surprisingly dramatic. However, some men may need professional help with this process.

The same thing applies to coming to terms with the fact that a man may not like his children very much when they grow up. He may not find them very nice persons and this requires real grief too. This *mea culpa* is all very well, but in the end he needs to grieve a straightforward sense of loss. But coming to terms with feelings about one's children is very difficult for a man, particularly from the affluent middle class. Th chances are that he will retreat into heavy drinking where he has a sanction from society provided that he doesn't become an alcoholic.

As there is minimal or no sanction for a man to grieve in our society there is also neither one for him to grow old. There is such a worship of youth that it is almost a social crime to grow old. Certainly this is true of the U.S.A. In an age of technology it has become very downgraded to have experience and wisdom. It is really passé, and, as a society, we shall have to pay a very high price for that, if not now, certainly later on.

As a society we compound all these problems for ourselves by living in an ethos (worshipping youth and technology) that says, "After 40 you've had it". We already throw the aged on the rubbish heap, so to speak; and now we are looking for the middle aged to throw. That is the threat that hangs over so many men. If his basic foundation has been weakened by strong feelings of personal deprivation and rejection, modern society's turndown is all the harsher to bear.

Fear of the rubbish heap is truly one of the important symptoms of the male menopause. Earlier we said that the terminology might appear ludicrous, but we trust by now the reader will be able to see some of the justification that clings to an uncomfortable, uncomplimentary, but in spite of, or because of those very qualities also, an illuminating, descriptive and near-definitive phrase. For us, and we hope for the reader, it carries the ring of the over and/or under-active crisis that can overtake men in their middle years and consume them with bewilderment, insecurity, inadequacy, confusion and panic.

2 From the outside...looking in

It goes tick-tick, it's quieter than your heart beat, but it's slow dynamite, a gradual explosion, blasting the world we lived in to burnt-out pieces . . . Time . . . Gnaws away, and like a rat gnaws off its own foot caught in a trap, and then, with its foot gnawed off and the rat set free, couldn't run, couldn't go, bled and died . . .

Tennessee Williams *Sweet Bird of Youth*

Onlookers are not slow to spot a man in the throes of a menopausal trauma. We found it totally right and proper and not without a high degree of poetic symbolism that the artist John Bratby should have chosen two men who figured largely in the socio-politico scene during our early work on this book to represent the male menopause. His portrait of the MP John Stonehouse and the missing Lord Lucan was featured in a centre spread in the Daily Mirror. (Interestingly enough, Mrs Stonehouse herself said of her husband, "John seemed to become increasingly bad-tempered. This was most unlike him. But I put it down to general worries and maybe even his age. He was 49. There'd been a lot of talk about the male menopause. Maybe he was going through that . . .")

With Bratby, it may have been the artist's perception of the 'dog beneath the skin' that led him to view the victims that way. It may have been that he recognised only too quickly what was happening to him in the personae of others. Or it may have been both. T S Eliot clearly had this factor in mind when he wrote *The Family Reunion*.

Eliot is undoubtedly a candidate for the post of Poet of the Menopause, only rivalled perhaps by Gerard Manley Hopkins. From his earliest poems onwards, Eliot reflects the quintessential condition of the menopausal experience. The extract on p.11, taken from *The Love Song of J. Alfred Prufrock*, was written when he was 29.

The following extract, from *The Dry Salvages,* came in 1935 when he was 47.

> Trying to unweave, unwind, unravel
> And piece together the past and the future,
> Between midnight and dawn, when the past is all deception,
> The future futureless, before the morning watch
> When time stops and time is never ending;

And from *The Hollow Men* comes this encapsulated concept:

> Between the potency
> And the existence . . .
> Falls the Shadow
>
> . . .
>
> *This is the way the world ends*
> *Not with a bang but a whimper.*

The idea of ending 'not with a bang but a whimper' is truly menopausal — at whatever level the line is interpreted — as is, from the same poem, the baleful cry, "Here we go round the prickly pear at five o'clock in the morning".

Turning to a different mode of poetic expression we find the following sonnet by Manley Hopkins also to scream *sotto voce* with a typically menopausal SOS:

> Justus quidem tu es, Domine, si disputem tecum: verum tamen
>   justa loquar ad te: Quare via impiorum prosperatur? Ec.
>
> Thou art indeed just, Lord, if I contend
> With thee; but, sir, so what I plead is just.
> Why do sinners' ways prosper? and why must
> Disappointment all I endeavour end?
>   Wert thou my enemy, O thou my friend,
> How wouldst thou worse, I wonder, than thou dost'
> Defeat, thwart me? Oh, the sots and thralls of lust
> Do in spare hours more thrive than I that spend,
> Sir, life upon thy cause. See, banks and brakes
> Now, leavèd how thick! lacèd they are again
> With fretty chervil, look, and fresh wind shakes
> Them; birds build — but not I build; no, but strain,
> Time's eunuch, and not breed one work that wakes,
> Mine, O thou lord of life, send my roots rain.

It is not without significance that Hopkins was halfway into Education and The Church; the first a breeding ground for the condition and the second an apparent refuge. Here is an extract from a letter Hopkins wrote to Robert Bridges when they were both 41:

I must write something, though not so much as I have to say. The long delay was due to work, worry, and languishment of body and mind — which must be and will be; and indeed to diagnose my own case (for every man by forty is his own physician or a fool, they say; and yet again he who is his own physician has a fool for his patient — a form of epigram, by the bye, which, if you examine it, has a bad flaw), well then to judge of my case, I think that my fits of sadness, though they do not affect my judgement, resemble madness. Change is the only relief, and that I can seldom get.

Moving from poetry to drama there are one or two very striking examples of the menopausal male in action. Crispin, the central character of John Mortimer's *Collect Your Hand Baggage* seems to be an archetype. This is how he is introduced to us on his arrival at the waiting-room at London Airport where the play is set. "CRISPIN arrives with his friends. His arrival is noisy and somehow grand. CRISPIN himself is a middle-aged Bohemian with thin, blowing hair and a big tweed overcoat hanging open like a cloak. His grey flannel trousers have the air of having been slept in, his brown, rubber-soled shoes are cracked, and for long periods of the play a yellowing cigarette hangs from his bottom lip. In contrast, his friends are very young, very good-looking and well cared for."

Like the type mentioned on p.22 , Crispin does not go in for trendy gear, but contents himself by sporting the symbol of his peacock spirit. For them it was the (probably Tyrolean!) hat; for Crispin it is his affectation of the coat-as-cloak. The play is made up of variations on the plaintive theme of the middle-aged man's search for what he is not quite sure of — through associations with younger people; through his falsely perceived sexual attractiveness to his land-lady's young daughter; and through his immature assessment of his failing marriage.

Another play based on the archetypal menopausal man is Robert Bolt's *Flowering Cherry* in which we have a central character who moves from one typical symptom to another during the course of the action. He never talks about himself as if he were menopausal. He has no need to. All his actions add up to a complete portrait. There is the boasting, the fantasy, the memory of things past, the falling for a young girl, the jealousy and resentment of his grown son, the futile dramatic gestures and the total retreat from reality. Bolt describes him like this: "CHERRY is a burly man of about fifty with a round red face and thinning grey hair. His carriage is confident, his expression heavy, but there is about the eyes and mouth the sadness and confusion of the immature. His clothes are good and timidly sportif, of earth colours, and include a trilby turned down back and front and a fawn waistcoat with leather buttons."

From a different world entirely comes the figure of Leo Harting, the central character in John Le Carré's *A Small Town in Germany* (Heinemann). It seems possible that Leo has defected from his post at the British Embassy, and Turner is brought in to investigate. Here he is talking with Bradford, Leo's superior officer. Bradford is speaking:

'So far as anyone knows, he has no woman. Does that satisfy you?'
'Perhaps he's queer.'
'I'm sure he's nothing of the sort.'
'It's broken out in him. We're all a bit mad, aren't we, round about
    our age? The male menopause, how about that?'
'That is an absurd suggestion.'
'Is it?'
'To the best of my knowledge, yes.' Bradfield's voice was trembling
    with anger; Turner's barely rose above a murmur.
'We never know though, do we? Not till it's too late.'

Later, Turner makes this assessment: "He didn't screw around. He wasn't queer. He'd no friends, but he wasn't a recluse. He never stole money, he played the organ in Chapel, took a certain interest in his garden and loved his neighbour as himself. Is that it? He wasn't any bloody thing, positive or negative. What was he then, for Christ's sake: The Embassy Eunuch?" (Shades of Hopkins)

. . . he didn't like fakes any more; he wanted the truth. The male menopause: that is it. He was disgusted with himself . . . for what he'd failed to do, sins of omission . . . signs of commission. We all know that feeling, don't we? Well, Leo had it. In full measure. So he decided to get what he was owed . . .

Robert Bolt's Cherry rebelled — and it cost him his life. John Le Carré's Leo also rebelled and paid the same price, although in much more sinister circumstances since it is a 'spy' story.

To end this menopausal gallery, drawn from fiction, there is the character of Ivan Ivanovich Ivanov from Anton Tchekov's play, *Ivanov*. There are two factors that make this character study of special interest to us. Firstly, Tchekov was a doctor of medicine. Secondly, he was 27 when he wrote the play (1887) and was living in a Russia as menopausal and as threatened as is Britain in the 70's. Tchekov's *Ivanov* (the Russian equivalent of our Everyman or Man in the Street) has all the symptoms — and he talks about them. We see him with his doctor, complaining of the physical symptoms. He finds no hope in his marital situation. He is cynical about the possibility of his loving a young woman who admires and desires him. But, true to form, a little later he thinks his salvation is to be found in her arms. And even truer to form, shortly

after he decides that even that is hopeless and is overcome by doubts
and misgivings. Here he is at the end of the play, calling off his wedding
to Sasha, the girl in question, and trying to explain what is happening
to him.

IVANOV I won't try to explain to you what sort of person I am —
whether I'm honest or base, healthy or mentally sick. You wouldn't
grasp it. I used to be young, eager, sincere and intelligent. I used to
love, hate and believe in my own way, differently from other people;
I used to work like ten men, and hope like ten men, too; I fought wind-
mills, I tried to ram down walls with my head . . . Without realizing
my strength or weakness, without reasoning, without knowing anything
about life, I took up a burden which promptly tore my muscles and
broke my back; I went all out to spend myself, I got drunk, I got
excited, I worked madly, I did everything without moderation. Well,
what else could I do. There are so few of us, there's so much work to be
done, so much! God, how much! And now how cruelly life, the life
which I fought against, is avenging itself on me. I've worn myself out.
At thirty-five I feel like a man after a drunken bout, I'm old already, I've
put on an old man's dressing-gown. I go about with a heavy head, with
a lazy soul, tired and broken, without faith, without love, without
aim; I wander about among my friends like a shadow, and I don't
know who I am, or why I live, or what I want. Already it seems to me
that love is silly, that caresses and endearments are sugary nonsense,
that there isn't any meaning in work, that song and impassioned words
are trivial and old-fashioned. And wherever I go, I bring misery, blank
boredom, discontent, disgust with life . . . I'm ruined, hopelessly
ruined! Before you stands a man tired at thirty-five, disenchanted,
crushed by his trivial efforts — burning with shame and jeering at his
own weakness . . . Oh, how my pride revolts. I feel suffocated with
anger! I've been going down hill long enough, now I'm going to stop!
There's a limit to everything! Stand away! Thank you, Sasha!
SASHA [shrieks]. Nikolai, for God's sake! Stop him!
IVANOV. Leave me alone! [Runs aside and shoots himself.]

It would be hardly fair or proper to leave poetry and drama without
mentioning that in the Seven Ages of Man speech in *As You Like It*,
Shakespeare offers no candidate. His fifth and sixth stages, which
presumably are the relevant ones, are the "justice, in fair round belly
with good capon lin'd" and "the lean and slipper'd pantaloon, with
spectacles on nose and pouch on side". However, Shakespeare's
vacuum, for his times, is more than filled by Milton who, in *Paradise
Lost*, offers us the following concentrate: "Demoniac frenzy, moping
melancholy, and moon-struck madness" — surely that condition will
suffice since it even brings in the guns of meno-lunar cycles.

Whether in fact or fiction, prose, poetry or drama, the victim of the male menopause is seldom seen as a suitable case for sympathetic treatment. He usually invites ridicule or rejection — and more often than not gets both. In particular he asks for them when involved in one of the all-too-familiar infatuations that show the seemingly phallic tip of the total middle-age iceberg. (There is an analogy here in that the ice-cold grip of frigidity prevents warm, loving relationships from being made. Just as the nymphomaniac may be manifesting a real, inner frigidity, so may the frantic, groping chaser of girls. The male is worse off in one feature only: his failure to be able to enter fully into a warm, mature sexual relationship can be seen to be so in the non-erect penis that is an emblem of his drooping spirit.)

The irresistible desire of many of the men to touch, pat, tickle and pinch the bodies of young girls, or even the less objectionable cuddling and putting of arms round shoulders, can and frequently does lead to uncomfortable social situations. Sometimes the inter-action goes no further than the man making his 'play' and the girl, good-humouredly or resentfully, tolerating it — or telling him to get lost, facetiously or cuttingly. Sometimes the rebuff will bring the man to halt in his tracks — to see himself in a truer light than before — and this can be therapeutic, but a rebuff at this stage can also be much more painful to him than in his youth and it can also make his situation worse. Should this occur, it could result in an ugly scene with the man attempting to recover his lost 'face' by putting the girl down; or with him rushing off even more frantically after further possibilities of conquests.

If the man is not rejected, there will be a strong possibility that an affaire will develop — with the man being much more smitten than the girl. True, she may be flattered, but he will float off on to Cloud Nine — transported from mundane, middle-aged, middle management into ecstasies.

Some girls really fall for the man, since, in spite of the menopausal overtones, older men are attractive — just because of their age — to some young women. There is also the plain magnetism of the man's 'status' (often seen by the young woman as a form of real power) and the affluent life style he will be able to present.

Some girls, and they seem to be in the majority, will merely enjoy what appeals to them while the generosity, and sometimes prodigality, of the first flush lasts. He will then be exploited for all the meals, nights out, clothes and expensive gifts that can be painlessly extracted. When the reckoning comes, the man in this situation will find that what was at first a transport of delight has only too quickly shown itself to be no more than a vehicle in which he was taken for a ride.

There are other girls too who find the menopausal male attractive because of his condition. Their psychological attitude is complex — and not likely to do him much good, they are probably looking for a combination of father figure and infant son, and his apparently helpless state ("But it's not his fault, poor thing") appeals to their personality inadequacies and their immature emotional needs.

Perhaps the most unattractive cases in this area are to be found among those men who are so unsure of themselves that they can only rely on the weapons of position and affluence to convince themselves they can attract women. This is sad enough on its own account, but we have in mind those men who do not in fact possess the attributes they feel they need. They are in a terrible position — frustrated and bitter — and many of them are tempted to the rather sordid middle class crimes of defaulting with funds or executing petty forgeries.

Not all cases of men's menopausal 'sexual' explosions end in disaster or court proceedings — at least of the criminal kind. We have two cases now that offer contrasting perspectives of the menopausal man/young girl category. They are both given as personal statements, and the first comes from M/s Joan Mackay who was separated from her husband when she talked to us at the beginning of our research. As we write now however, events have moved on and she is divorced from her husband. He has married the girl in question. M/s Mackay is now 48; her ex-husband, Donald is 52; and the girl is 20.

I think Donald's unrest — the stress, the strain, the depression and the going off the rails . . . all text book behaviour for the male menopause — began five to six years ago when our grandchild, Marcus, left with his mother to go to Australia. Donald absolutely adored him and when he was no longer there he retreated right into himself. We both came home and had a jolly good howl after seeing them off, but in Donald's case he didn't get over it. He withdrew completely and began to be very sick. He got depressed and started having all these pains so acutely that we had to go to see the doctor — a thing we hadn't done for years. The doctor said, "This is no good. You know, if you carry on like this you'll get an ulcer."

The baby had been with us for over a year and Donald adored him so, when he took it so badly, the only thing I could think of doing was to get the brochures to see when we could go and visit them. In the event that wasn't much help because Donald said just before we went, "I'd almost rather not be going. It will be marvellous to see them — but awful to leave. I don't think I shall be able to face it."

I think what happened was that he began to realise how much he depended upon young children — how much easier it was for him to communicate with them than with the world outside. He didn't feel threatened by children. They would accept him for what he was without any sense of challenge. One of the parents at school has been heard to say, "Mr Mackay doesn't behave at all like he's 50. He's just one with all those youngsters." I think that is terribly pathetic in a grown man, but it all fits with trying to cling to youth by surrounding yourself with them and trying to recapture what you felt when you were a child.

Another key factor was the sense of stress and strain at school. Things weren't going as he wanted them by any means. Donald didn't tell me. I had to discover it for myself because he wasn't the kind of person to talk openly and discuss things, particularly if they were going wrong. It was one of the senior members of the school staff who said, "I thought at the last staff meeting that he was a sick man. I was worried about him. He seemed to be under great strain."

He always was a reserved person but now it became worse. Many years ago it was a joke — he was so secretive that his right hand didn't know what his left was doing — but as he got older it became pathetic. He would sit every night watching television — unless he had a meeting — sucking his thumb. It was always his thumb knuckle. There was a permanent mark there from the habit.

Once or twice when I've been watching television with him — and knitting — I've looked at him and realised that he was just not seeing the screen. Then he'd see me watching him and say, "What's the matter? What are you looking at? Why are you watching me?" Then, of course, I'd say, "Oh nothing," and I suppose in that kind of way we ceased to communicate — even the little we had done previously. That meant he had no-one to communicate with at all since he only really related with me. Of course, he was loth to admit that he was deeply worried about failing since I do the same sort of job — but I get on very well with my staff at the personal level. They come round for coffee and that kind of thing — and he knew he couldn't get that relationship going with his staff. He was interested in the children at school but not the people he worked with, not at a human level. Real human problems are things he's shied away from, even with his own children. It was fine while they were very young — he was a model father — but once they were like people he couldn't communicate with them. I suppose he needed all his relationships to be unrealistic, unchallenging and non-demanding. This is what he will be getting from his liaison with this girl. She won't be making any demands while their affaire is in its early stages and he won't talk to her about problems in education or anything to do with his work. He would just chop reality out of his life with her — cut it all down and forget about the real world.

I didn't know about the girl until after he'd left. It all came about in such an apparently insignificant way really — stupid thing. There had been some post for him, but instead of opening it he put it in his pocket and disappeared with it. Later that evening I said, "Who was the letter from?" He said, "None of your business." I said, "Oh come on; who are you getting letters from that I shouldn't know about?" and he said, "It's nothing to do with you." I rather kept on about it because I thought it was funny. And then, suddenly, all hell broke loose. He walked up and down the bedroom and stormed and ranted and raved about interfering and this, that and the other. I said, "I've no desire to interfere. I always leave my letters around." Then out of the blue he turned to me: "If you really want to know; for the last three to four years I would far rather have been on my own."

It was just like someone giving you one in the solar plexus because we'd been on marvellous holidays and done everything together and I had no inkling he felt like that. I just sort of crumpled and he went off to sleep in the other bedroom. He did the same thing the next night, but I didn't get to sleep at all so, at six in the morning, I woke him up because I felt we had to talk. He looked wretched just like a little lost boy who you couldn't get to help.

But he started to talk. He talked about not having done the things he wanted to, but he never said what they were. And then he started talking about dying. "I might die. I know you'll never understand this since you're not worried about death but I am. I'm absolutely petrified of dying and I'm just not doing things I need to for fulfilment before I die." And all this time he was holding on to my hands and pulling at me earnestly.

The next morning I felt much more relaxed. After all, we had communicated in a sort of way for the first time in years. We agreed that things were tense and that he was tired, so we put off talking any more until the next holiday in three weeks when we were going to Paris. He seemed a lot happier and I was obviously thinking he had sorted something out. Consequently, when the blow came it was much worse. If he'd left two or three days after the quarrel I could have understood it, but he was much nicer, much kinder — and we had better sex relations than we'd had for some time. I felt that it was all so dishonest. He'd strung me along and given me an unwarranted sense of security.

It was about a month after he'd gone that I found out he was with this girl. At first, I felt very sorry for him — after getting over the shock of his brief letter telling me he was not coming home one night. I used to think of him all alone in a bed-sit or a hotel. I even put things together for him in his cardboard box. I mean, he'd said he needed to be on his own to try and work out how to make a life for himself that was more meaningful than it had been before. Then, quite by chance, one of the mothers at his school happened to say, "I'm terribly sorry about your husband, of course, but isn't he supposed to be living with A. . C. . . . . .?" And all that time I had been worried about him being suicidal. I'd even thought of ringing the police and asking if anybody had been found.

I think he must have been sexually attracted to her for some time. And there's where the searching for lost youth comes up again, because in many ways she's just like I was when we first met. I did look like her . . . had long hair, did sing and act. It is the classic case of falling for the girl who is like the wife, except that I'm quite slim now and she is a busty type girl with high cheekbones and a fat face. But there is no doubt that in many ways she is a younger version of me, except that I don't like to think I'm the same sort of person that she is basically.

Donald would never admit it of course but he is searching for something that will take him back. He's using her younger face to hide behind so that he doesn't have to see his own. Kidding himself that he's young again. It probably came to him that his work at school wasn't good enough — that he wasn't getting anything out of it — and, on top of that, what did he have at home? He had a wife who wasn't dependent upon him physically or financially. I may have been emotionally, but I certainly wasn't the 'little woman at home'. Many people have suggested that he might have found me a threat because I was successful and he wasn't — and instead of launching out and doing something about it, it just made him feel all the more inadequate. Actually, during that long talk he said "You could run my school much better than I can. You could get the staff working better for you than I can."

And I suppose that that sort of feeling pervaded our relationship from the beginning. Ever since we set up home together twenty seven years ago I've always organised everything. Although we've always done things together I made all the arrangements. I sometimes wished he would go off on his own and just do something, but he would always rely on me and tag on. I encouraged him to take a year off from school. I said, "Why don't you go to the Education Office and tell them that you've reached saturation point and need a longish leave of absence?" I was sure if they knew the bad state he was in they would have been co-operative. It would have given him a chance to stand on his own and me a chance to find out what it might be like to be alone after all those years. He'd been in education ever since he left Oxford and he thought he'd never seen the other half of life, people or the world. He knew he was stuck, but was too arrogant to admit it. He had to run away from his sense of failure by going off with this young girl.

He didn't even learn when his father died. Now I'm sure that a man's father dying has a lot to do with the effect of a man's menopause, and Donald couldn't face visiting him when he was sick — he was that afraid of death. But when his younger brother was made the executor he didn't understand that his father had known all along that he was hopeless in business things — anything to do with the real world. That should have got through to him but it didn't. He hated all the admin and business side of his work. Every school he's left found many pieces of admin for someone else to clear up. Anything from the real world makes him withdraw.

Another example happened when I had a telegram from the Foreign

Office saying to ring them urgently. Our elder daughter had been involved in a shooting incident outside Karachi. She had been shot twice in the leg and her husband had been killed. Christine, our daughter, was being flown back to Heathrow and we were needed to meet her there. I went to his school and showed him the telegram. I told him Christine's husband had been killed and everything. All he did was to sit behind his desk and say, "What am I supposed to do?" and for the first time I lost my temper. I told him exactly what I thought of him. He went ashen white and just sat there clasping the sides of his desk with his knuckles all white. But didn't do or say a thing.

After all this it's difficult to know why I didn't see it all before, but having once seen it I don't think I'd want to live with him again. It's not a case of stopping loving someone but being realistic about what's happening — and by that very standard, I don't think he would want to come back if the affaire with the girl broke up. For one thing he'd be too arrogant to admit he'd made a mistake and for another he'd go back to his mother and their housekeeper where everyone would say he was marvellous and that everything he did was wonderful. It would be interesting to know though how they would take him having dyed his hair and he's let it grow much longer just to look younger!

In a sense, he's done me a favour. If he was going to have nervous breakdowns, and things like that, I would have had an awful life. Since he became riddled with so many insecurities I think it's better that he did go off with the girl otherwise I might have tried all kinds of rescues and I would have been worse off again. I feel in many ways now that he was a restricting influence on me although he would never have thought it and neither would I. But you do tend to tailor yourself to what you think is required of you. And I think now, "Look where it got me," so I can feel now that it was a good thing — although it was grim while it was happening and Donald obviously went through a very bad time. But, as one of my close friends said who hadn't seen me for a year or so, "You know you're not the same person that you were a year ago. You just don't resemble that person. Your appearance is different to start with and psychologically it's just as if you've been liberated. You were very much the headmaster's wife before, doing all the things that were expected of you."

I doubt if Donald would recognise me now. I have lost four stones in weight. I wear quite different clothes now, and I also have a series of wigs. I feel that I can get on with living again and leave Donald's future to him. After all the traumas I'm more concerned about my own development and my own future. It's just being realistic and coming to terms with what has happened — sad as it may be.

Our next case has some similarity with that of Joan and Donald

Mackay — but the resolution of the crisis and the resolutions that have emerged from it are in marked contrast. This time the testimony comes from the man. He has asked us not to reveal his identity.

I was married when I was 21. Joanna, my wife, was 17. We shared the traditional attitudes to sexual relationships: being in love, getting married — the whole thing. I was completely faithful for 10 years with very little strain. Then, one night at an office party, I began to get on very well with a secretary to whom I had been enormously attracted for some time. I ended up sleeping with her and that was the beginning of a three week passionate affaire. It might have gone on for much longer, but I realised that unless I put an end to it fairly smartly I would get into water too deep for me and, at that time, I could see only too clearly that it was ridiculous to jeopardise my marriage. That was when I was about 30.

By the time I was 40 I began to see things in a different light. I began to notice my receding hairline far too often — and then to experience the unpleasantness of a growing paunch. I thought, "In five years no other woman will want to sleep with me — even if they do now."

But it wasn't just a sexual thing. It was everything in my life. I looked around and found there was no area in which I could find cause for hope. I had been overlooked for promotion at work, and the job had been given to a man seven years younger. There was the dawning of under-standing that I was never going to get right to the top. I'm not a failure — but I'm certainly no great success. But now I am more resigned to what really is and I don't feel the need to over-respond as I did then. That was about five years ago.

I met this woman who was five years younger than my wife and we used to go out very late together, dancing and nightclubbing. She was unhappily married and had an arrangement with her husband so it didn't matter if she arrived home at four in the morning. Her husband didn't ask any questions and neither did my wife — but for entirely different reasons. I had already started to stay out far too late, drinking my problems away, so she was used to it.

I never slept with this woman because we had nowhere to go and I'm not the sort who can book a hotel and think, "Tonight's the night." For me, it has to be spontaneous or not at all. In the end we just drifted apart, but I found the idea of bolstering my ego and flagging self-image, with another woman, very appealing. So, I met another woman on a business trip and we slept together and had a very good time, but although I wanted to keep it going when we got back to England, she didn't — so that was that.

Then, drink again. At another office party one of the sectretaries got very drunk and I was well on my way so, when someone said, "Why don't you two go out and get something to eat?'' — we did, and that was that again but in a different way because an affaire very quickly grew out of it. It was a bad move. Everyone in the office started talking and they had plenty to talk about. She rang one day from Finland, drunk and so loud over the phone that almost everybody could overhear. That struck me as being very childish on her part — so terribly childish that I was a bit sickened. Later she wrote me a letter couched in the same childish-to-drunk tones and that really convinced me. However, before she returned from Finland I met another girl, Sharon, and once again, that was that. Within three days I was madly in love with her. It wasn't just sex, I was completely euphoric about her, about me and about the world at large. We spent whole evenings together without rushing to get back to bed and they actually did fly.

Then I started staying with her all night. She had a flat and I told my wife I was staying with a man friend with whom I had occasionally spent the night when work was heavy. Sex was important though — the old chemistry thing really worked with Sharon, and before I knew it I was building a total fantasy world on the basis of my relationship with this 21 year old girl. By this time, the women having progressively got younger, she really was young enough to be my daughter. Although she was only 21 she was mature beyond her years and I became thoroughly infatuated, and, for her part, she had told her parents about me even before we'd slept together. Then we did sleep together and she told them about that too but I was too euphoric to complain — even when they said they wanted to meet me! I felt that good, I knew I could cope with anything.

After a time they took her on holiday to Greece hoping it might prove a cooling-off time. It did, in fact, and the whole affaire broke up after that. But it wasn't just the holiday nor the predictable warnings from parents. Other things had begun to creep up from my side. At first Sharon just wanted me to tell my wife about her. Then she wanted me to leave my wife and finally, of course, she wanted me to marry her. The progression was, I suppose, inevitable. I had realised it was lonely for her when I went home at week-ends, but I insisted on doing that — I felt I owed it to my wife anyway. I wanted to keep up appearances, and I wanted to be with our three children. But Sharon kept up the pressure and towards the end she really laid it on. If only you could have affaires with girls who realise you aren't going to leave your wife! But it doesn't work like that, so I began seriously to consider leaving Joanna . . . and the prospect looked very bleak. I knew she would grab every penny she could and that would leave me badly off and although I could have fought her over the money she would have claimed half the goods. Then there was the awful guilt about never being able to repay her for what she had done in making the family — the devotion she had shown to me and the children. But, more than anything, there was the fear that it wouldn't work with Sharon, because she would inevitably fall for a younger man as time went on — and where would that leave me? We approached the affaire from different positions. For her it was just a part of growing up but for me she was likely to become vitally necessary. She had a very promising career that would take her away from me, physically as well as psychologically, and that troubled me. Also, I still loved my wife. People weren't able to understand that, but you can't have a marriage that lasts for twenty two years without a very deep bond. There was something that had kept us together for all that time. I loved both women in fact and, what is more, needed both — one for all the richness of the past and the other for the promise of the future and the boost it gave to my ego.

Perhaps if I hadn't married so young I might not have run after women so much. Perhaps the crisis during those years might have expressed itself in different ways, but as it was, it was sex that was important with drink running a close second. Of course, male chauvinism was there as well; my wife had been a virgin when we met and that was very important to me, and if she had an affaire now I'd be terribly jealous — I'm a very jealous person and, as might be expected, I need security too. Joanna is a fantastically strong woman; much stronger in personality than I am and I found I needed her strength. She was gold, there was no doubt about it — and while Sharon too was gold, it was of a different sort. I felt if I had put them in the scales, my wife would weigh the more.

Actually my wife was very beautiful — and in a similar way to Sharon. So it was a case of history repeating itself but with a younger target so that I felt younger too. That is, until it came to sex. My wife was perfectly happy about sex until after our third child and then it became something of a wifely duty. That's slightly unfair, but I was the one to set the pace. I continued to make love with my wife during the time with Sharon to keep up the facade — and it wasn't too difficult since we made love once during the week and once at the week-end. But with Sharon as well, quite frankly I began to get jolly tired. I discovered that it took a lot of me. Things are different by the time you get to my age. Fortunately, my wife didn't mind or suspect. She was going through the menopause herself at the time and began to get more apathetic about sex.

Many people were concerned about me. Those who knew both of us wanted me to 'go back' to Joanna but others seemed to have a more open mind. As for me, I was quite calculating and worked out that Sharon would probably do my career good. She was intelligent, attractive and young and all men like to be seen with a girl like that. The boost in status I felt was good and real. But then people at the office started taking me to one side and warning me that I was making a fool of myself.

They made me think twice about what being adult means and I realised it wasn't on so I painted a very black picture to Sharon before she went to Greece explaining all the financial difficulties and the legal wrangles. Finally I said, "It's no good unless you're willing to give up everything for us including your career because it won't work if you're going off all the time." That really had an effect on her and was the thing that tipped the scales. So when I rang her in Greece and she sounded cold I knew that was it — although she did say her parents weren't pressurising her at all. In a strangely roundabout way it was Sharon's Greece trip that brought it all out in the open with my wife.

I was due to meet Sharon at her place and needed the car. My wife wanted it to do the shopping. She asked why I wanted it and I said "Business" and that it would be better not to discuss it any further. That did it. I suppose I must have known it would and many of my friends said later that I was subconsciously willing it to a head. Anyway, she said, "That's it. I've had enough. I've had a real bellyfull and I'm not standing it a moment longer. We'll stay up all night if necessary, but you are going to tell me everything: I want to know her name, her age, how many times you've slept with her and whether you're staying here or going."

I answered her completely honestly — or as honestly as I could without hurting her feelings too much, although I suspect there was also an element of straightforward cowardice in it as well.

My wife insisted on having the car. She dropped me at the office and said that if I didn't come home that night she didn't want to see me again. It didn't matter how late so long as I returned otherwise it was all over. So I met Sharon as we'd agreed and it was all very civilised. We went for a meal and talked things over, coming to the conclusion that it was hopeless. We went back to her flat and there were lots of tears, but we both knew for sure that it had come to an end. We were both still attracted to each other as before, and indeed later a friend brought us together in a bar, and it was the same thing still — but just too painful and upsetting. So I went back to my wife and didn't regret it. Of course, it was rough at first because she kept having a go at me, saying that I had ruined her life by destroying her trust in me. I know it will take a long time to win that back but I am trying. Nothing dramatic — I've seen how destructive the big dramatic things can be. I am being genuinely affectionate and trying to rebuild the fondness there once had been. One day though she went on so much that eventually I said, "I can't stand this any more. There is no point in going on with the marriage if it's going to be like this for ever. There's no purpose in staying." She said she wouldn't mention it again and she has kept her word.

My hope is that, in the long run, the incident of Sharon — the highlight and symbol of my crisis as it were — will even strengthen my marriage. It certainly made me appreciate my wife more when I had to weigh up her virtues against Sharon's. Also, I had to re-assess what I was looking for in life: what was realistic, what was possible and what was an over-response to frustration. Had I been sure I could have started again with Sharon I might have gone with her and what she stood for: fresh beginnings, fresh families, fresh money problems — all the hopes and fears, challenges, opportunities and threats of youth. Taking on all that when you're nearly 46 is very difficult. So, although the affaires, the rebellion if you like, did rejuvenate me and I felt marvellous while things were going well, in the final resort I settled down to realising the significance of the word 'pension' — and that means coming to terms with a lot of things. Having done so, far from being unhappy, unfulfilled or frustrated, on the contrary I'm really quite happy, so the mid-life crisis might have done good in spite of all its sting.

Wives and families are obviously special cases — they see the menopausal man 'from the outside . . . looking in', and just as life can be made difficult for the spouse and family if the woman experiences a bad menopause — so can the wife suffer when the man falls victim to an unhappy time. And from the men and their families we have spoken to we know that this 'unhappy time' can last from weeks and months to four to five years.

If the man displays symptoms of depression as the first signs these can be difficult to detect — as they can in most cases of depression — until they assume proportions that make it difficult to know how to respond. At first they may seem like normal responses to specific stresses at work or in the family and the escalation may be so gradual that the whole family may be enmeshed before anyone realises that the mood swings are abnormal. When this has occurred it can be difficult to allocate with any accuracy first causes — or to separate them from symptoms.

If the man makes drastic changes in his drinking or dressing habits, or begins to stay out late with an accumulation of implausible excuses, it is easier for the family to detect what might be happening. But it is still no easier to respond in a manner that will bring positive results since the last thing the menopausal family man wants is to be challenged.

The timing of the man's crisis may be unfortunate in the extreme. His wife may be trying to work through her own menopause; the children may have left and there are, therefore, new inter-actions to be discovered between the two of them; or the children may be progressing their equally unsteady way through their valid, 'first' adolescences. When such a collection of possibly insecure people is trying to solve its problems it can be an almost impossible task for them to help sort each other out as well. Sometimes the recognition of crises in other members of the family can help to create heightened awareness and deeper understanding, and we have had such cases described to us; but the general pattern is one of a failure to understand, an inability to read signals accurately or to perceive change until it is too late in the day, and there is a growing confusion about the acts and motives of people who all thought they 'knew' each other.

Possibly, open discussion with frank self-disclosure about each individual's inner state would go a long way to healing the situation and those involved in it. But hot flushes, middle-aged spread (physical and psychological), barrenness and impotence are not factors conducive to relaxed discussion about personal relationships. And even in families where the adolescent children have not experienced any particular *sturm und drang* the simple change from their needing, wanting and admiring their parents to questioning (even mildly) their views, values and attitudes may be unbearable if the parents are feeling bad about themselves and therefore least able to manage even the slightest challenge — especially if the father has previously been inclined to authoritarian paternalism . . . the kind of role that gets badly knocked in the male menopause.

We have heard from many women about the difficulties that wives and families face when the man in the family gets the condition. It is important to note here that the recognition of the condition and appellation of the male menopause by the man's wife and/or children brings into play another set of forces. It is one thing for a man to use the phrase — it is entirely different, and quite unpalatable for some men, when it is actually referred to in his own home. A proportion might be able to find comfort and solace in the thought that they are understood, but the majority tend to view it — at the time, if not later — as direct or tangential criticism. This circular double-think is one of the most difficult and elusive of the menopausal symptoms, making it almost impossible for a wife or children to help . . . or to win. Indeed, the phrases, "I don't know what to do for the best" and "I don't know how I ever managed to live through it", have been used to us on many occasions. Witness to this are the opening remarks in the first personal statement that follows. It comes from a 50 year old woman who prefers to remain anonymous. Over the months we have been talking with her she has still been trying to cope with the apparently insurmountable problems caused by her husband's menopause. Until recently she was dedicated to improving her husband's condition and to repairing the marriage. But as we write, we have heard from her that divorce proceedings are under way — and she is attempting to put the many years of disturbance behind her. However, to use her own words, "I still can't get to grips with it all emotionally. I can understand it intellectually . . . but I am afraid that it is going to be a long time before it makes any kind of sense emotionally."

As you read this testimony, you may consider the possibility that the husband succumbed to an emotional or mental state that ought to be called disturbed or abnormal (and indeed one of the authorities to whom we regularly turned suggested that he was more psychopathic than menopausal) but the wife and her husband — as well as most of the people they turned to — are convinced it is an extreme case of a man suffering from the menopause.

Many people say to me, "I don't know how you stand it," or, "Why do you go on loving him?" or, "Why don't you leave him for good?" and the reason is that I feel he needs me so desperately. I don't know why I feel this so strongly but although he keeps pushing me away I think he does need me.

Now, of course, this may be because I want to feel this. I've always thought that love and patience don't go well together, but with him it's different somehow. In most things I'm very impatient. I can't wait for a letter in the post. If something is going to happen then I want to know about it. But for the past four years I have waited patiently. Every time he has said he will phone on a certain day I just live for that minute. And then when it comes he will only give me time for a sentence or two. I suppose it will have to stop really. For example, the doctor I saw the other day was very quick to say so. She's devoted her life to helping people in these difficult situations although she's only an ordinary GP. Actually she saw me privately because I'd been recommended to her — in her own home and without charging. She knows that most doctors have no time for this sort of thing so she was especially good and kind. She said, "You're in a state of breakdown. You can't go on like this. You must tell him that you're going to divorce him." I said, "I think that's just what he wants," and she said straight away, "No, I don't think it's what he wants at all." And that about sums up what is happening: conflict and contradiction. He *says* one thing and means another. I *think* one set of things yet feel quite differently . . . and it's been going on for well over 10 years.

He thinks that once he's out of the close confines of marriage we'll be the best of friends. We tried to sort out this ambiguous state very early on when he first showed signs of having his menopause and our doctor suggested that we should go to a psychiatrist. We both went at first but it was very expensive and in the end, when I went by myself, he advised me just to give up because there was no way of overcoming it. That's the way the children think as well. They want me to get out of it. But it's very difficult when I know he's suffering such great strain.

A little while ago he said he was afraid of me — that I had become a threat. So I became very meek and at that time he would ring up and arrange to see me at a certain time and whereas in the past he would never have bothered if he'd been three to four hours late. He used to ring to say, "I'm on my way — sorry to be late," and he'd do that every half hour or so. Before, I would have been fed up and said, "Oh hell, I've been cooking all day and you've ruined it," but then I thought, "Well, he's really trying." So there were no rows — because he thought he was doing what I wanted him to do.

Then it all came to a head and he said he had always done only what I had wanted of him. He saw the past in terms of living his life the way I wanted him to live it, whereas I thought it was a case of a family having responsibilities and the mother being the proper candidate for organising things. I mean, if you go and sit on the sand it's not because you want to make sand-castles, it's because you're on holiday and that's what you do if you have children. But twenty years after I suppose he thought, "My God, I've done all the things *she* wanted to do." But they weren't the things I wanted to do either.

When he started to re-assess things he said, "I'm 45 and I'm not living." I remember he said that again, later: "My God, I'm 50 and it's now or never." He tried to make excuses for himself but he got to the stage where there were none left and that's what happens to men and women alike when they get to the change. That's what the menopause is all about. They start to go off the rails and do all the things they've never done before and it gets out of hand. It runs away with them. The fact that he thought he'd lived a very closed and restricted life, always told what to do and never free made it bad when he tried to find a bit of freedom. It ran away with him and frightened him and got him into such difficulties. It was rather like when you have a teenage daughter who's been brought up very strictly. When she becomes 18 and you let her do what she likes, she's not capable of dealing with life — and he went off just like an adolescent off the string, completely irresponsible. He just didn't care what the children or I thought or felt. They, the children, have shut themselves off from him. They don't want to know. They don't want to know *him* and they won't discuss it with *me.*

It's the selfishness of what my husband's doing that is completely callous and cruel. He has seen me in terrible distress and my legs have buckled under me so that I was in a state of complete collapse because of his cruelty — and he was never like it before. But on the other hand, I don't honestly think that he knows what he's doing. He can't do. His disposition has changed so much. He's become obsessed with holding his job — just hanging on — yet at the same time he has megalomaniac urges to get to the top and beat everybody else.

I suppose it first started when he was about 38 — just over fifteen years ago. The firm he had originally worked for when he came out of the forces was taken over and became a computerised, cut-throat operation and my husband was threatened and attracted at one and the same time. I think he thought he was having a good time. OK; if I'm married to a man who meets a woman and sleeps with her and I don't know about it, I wouldn't think any the worse of him. I think this is life. I think a man who is just so good all through his married life that he says, "I've never been unfaithful to my wife," . . . well, I'd say, "Poor fellow."

I did meet one man myself after all my husband's trouble started. I was attracted to him — but I found I was being attracted by all the problems that my husband had. He had the same background, the same kind of job. He looked like him, behaved like him and was completely unreliable like him. What is more he was impotent like my husband. Eventually he did go back to his wife — his second — and treated her in the same way. I'm sure he was menopausal too.

Occasionally I wish I could meet someone now — but I just don't. It would have to be an executive or a surveyor or a solicitor or an architect; somebody in that type of job. Somebody who speaks reasonably well and knows his wines when he takes you dining. I don't want to go and have fish and chips. I'm not a loner. I need people. I'm a very warm affectionate person. I enjoy sex. I like it. I think it's very important — and all that side of life is being deprived me by my husband, the way he is. It even went so far that I didn't have any problem with my own menopause I was so busy concentrating on my husband's. I got through mine quite naturally and normally by comparison. He was rushing around everywhere trying to find something — I don't know what. He started living away from home or spending every night in a local pub, drinking till the early hours. I went with him once or twice but he complained that the other customers talked to me and not to him. He began to get paranoiac.

This is the trouble. As one of his work colleagues said, "When one thing starts to go — the lot goes. You lose confidence in yourself and work goes, sex goes, everything goes." But instead of getting down to it and finding out what was really the matter — getting some medical help to see him through the menopause — he went off the rails completely. It's very frightening really. He lives in an absolute dream world of his own, quite out of touch with reality. I gave him an article to read not long ago that described the unrealness of the state that menopausal men can get into. He recognised himself in it definitely — and I know he keeps on reading it. He's even commented upon the changes himself.

They were dramatic. We had been married for about fifteen years and had three children, and from being a kind, generous, willing, co-operative person he became uncooperative, cruel, greedy and selfish. From treating me as if I was everything to him he started to pull me down and be the exact opposite. Before we'd always agreed about him leaving the Services. Now he started to say it was all my fault and that he should have stayed and he would have had a fantastic career.

He began to go in for tremendous Walter Mitty ideas that things would have been different and he would have been on the top.

Suddenly all the mistakes we'd made were all my fault and he did nothing but look back on the mistakes and forgot all the good times. He began to build up the girls against me. Before he'd been full of praise to everybody about me and them, but when they were about 11 and 13 everything changed. He started to talk about them and only them. They were always right and he was proud of them — and I was always wrong. If they were rude to me, he would say they hadn't been. If I suggested they might tidy their room, he would rush up and do it for them. It made me feel very low. Now he says I was creating an atmosphere.

He had a good job at the time — in entertainment — and he said he had been given the sack because he'd been fooling about with another woman when they were on work projects, I'm sure that was only to give himself an ego boost sexually and to cover up for getting the sack. After that he told me many stories about other women — how he'd had affaires and they had got pregnant and there had been abortions. But I've never seen any sign of him being a womaniser. He didn't even seem capable of chatting up women and of course there had been his impotence problem during all these years anyway. I really don't believe a word of it — though of course it may be true. It's much more likely to be an ego boost for him and a put-down for me.

He was talking about one of these women once, so I said to him, "I don't want to take second place to anyone else. I couldn't bear to be in competition. I'm not in competition, am I?" He said, "Only perhaps with me." And I think that's true. He seems to have been trying to beat me all the time although the psychiatrist said, "She's not in competition with you, thank god!" I'm sure he thought of me as competition in bed as well.

I remember I once said to him, "Have you got a sexual problem?" because there had been the impotence. He said, "I've got a sexual prob lem; I've got a financial problem; and I've got a drink problem." He had too: sometimes he would go six months or a year without being interested in sex — and it was always me that instigated it.

Then it became different. I mean, you had only to go like that and he would have an erection . . . but he could never get rid of it, never get any relief. During sex, I used to say, "Oh relax for God's sake," and he'd say, "I am RELAXED!" He's said to me often since, "I'm no good to you. I can't even take you to bed. I think that if I did anyway, I might kill you." He has knocked me about twice, and that too is quite out of character from what he used to be. But he has changed so drastically. It's as though he is in the grip of something terrible and macabre and it really frightens me.

In the car sometimes he's cried — actually started weeping while he's been driving. He's taken his hands off the wheel and gone all purple in the face. I've had to say, "For goodness sake calm down. You'll have a stroke in a minute." He's had to get out of the car to walk up and down to keep calm. It's all sheer frustration. He never smiles or laughs and he has withdrawn entirely into himself. He never talks if he can help it. Almost everything has gone out of control. He's got terribly fat and into a bad shape — all posture gone. He no longer has any self-discipline over his eating or drinking and he's got greedy.

He still seems to work hard, but he's got to work twice as much as anybody else for the same results. I'm convinced he's terrified every day of his life; every time there's going to be any re-organisation; every time there's going to be a meeting that they are going to give him the push. He says about three or four times a month, "There's a big meeting. Don't know if I can 'phone you. They're going to have a big purge." He's frightened to take any time off or to go on holiday in case something happens behind his back. He feels that they are all scheming and he can't trust anybody. It was made much worse when all the others were made into full somethings or other at the office and he wasn't. This upset him greatly.

When you come to boil it all down it isn't that he hasn't done well because he has. I think he's done tremendously well bearing in mind his deprived background — children's home and all that. It's what he thinks of himself that's causing all the trouble. He feels a failure although in no way could he be described as one. He's so mixed up about every-thing. He's in a terrible state — doesn't know what to think about his job and doesn't know what to think about me. He has talked more and more about suicide — putting himself under a bus. He used to like little children but he never sees his grandchildren. He's even said himself, "People have said to me 'Why don't you love your children like they deserve?'" It's as though he's become so work-minded that everything else has suffered as a result — but without him getting anything out of work. It's all just a symptom of this terrible feeling of failure and inadequacy.

He has said that he feels dead — thinking and feeling nothing at all. And while he's talked about these supposed affaires, most of the time he's said he was absolutely alone and lonely. Nothing adds up for him. It's as though he's been living in a fantasy world for a few years, pretending that the sexual side hasn't packed up although everything else has done. It might be a last gasp of pride — hoping that there's one thing left that isn't on the way out. But I think it's quite hopeless. It's the real menopause at its worst.

The next case comes from another wife of the same age — about 50. Her story doesn't involve the unnerving behavioural abnormalities suggestive of a gross mental disorder of the last, but it does give some idea of what it feels like to live with a menopausal type who responds to his problem by becoming over-active in the sexual peacock role. As in the last case, the wife is supported by the children — in this case a son — and, again repeating the pattern, that support is of little help to the woman . . . or her husband.

We're Cockneys, my husband and I. We've made a lot of money by sheer hard work and have been a successful working pair with the handbag factory. And there are so few couples like Jack and I. What ever we had, it was never yours or his, it was always ours. Everything that was earned was always shared. We never had a secret — never in our lives. We had some bad times, like when the factory had to go into liquidation — that was bad for Jack. He never was a demonstrative man, something to do with his mother being so hard and possessive I think, but he sat down broken-hearted and cried like a baby. But we pawned everything and got started again, and had a very good business going soon afterwards. So seven years ago we thought we'd worked hard enough to retire and we shut the factory and went away. We went everywhere; Mexico, California, Hawaii — everywhere. It was the happiest six months of my life.

Then, when we got back — the very day — Jack became impotent. It was terrible. He had been all right on the trip — like a man of 20 — and then this. When it first happened, this not being able to make love, he used to talk to me about it because he thought it worried me — but it didn't, not then. It doesn't now — not the sex side of it — even though I was a very hot natured person all my life and knew how to make love. So, at first he used to talk about it, but time went by and he stopped talking about it — and that's when the changes started to come about.

His whole personality changed. He never was one to be all dressed up and now he dresses very young. He doesn't look as bad as he might because he's still very slim and has some nice hair, but he worries about getting old and wants to look young and be in young company. And exactly the same thing happened to my brother. He went impotent and then started to want to look young and to seek out younger people all the time. They just want young company all the way — it's like a drug to them — whether it's boys or girls. It's a boost to their ego and it helps them think they're not getting old. Well, I mean being impotent is a big thing to have taken away from a man in his 50's.

My husband dresses younger than our son. When he goes out he wears very wide trousers. Gets them all from the King's Road — and until this all started he hated dressing up. Now it has to be right up to the minute or he won't wear it. When platforms were in, he wore platforms. And then very wide ties with loud colours and patterns. If it wasn't for me he'd go out looking atrocious. But I say to him, "You can't wear that tie and shirt together. It's ridiculous." He even went out and bought a pair of dark glasses for seventy pounds. He doesn't need glasses but he thinks these make him look trendy. He also wears a toupee. He got that almost the minute the impotence set in. That was the first thing. He was slightly bald before, but he didn't mind. Now he wears this piece and combs his hair on the side. My son read the piece in the Sunday Times where it said they combed their hair on one side and he cut it out and sent it to me. "You'd never believe it," he said, "It's like reading about my own father. He does the lot." The change is so obvious — it's incredible. I actually showed him the article, hoping it might help him — and I think it would have done at the beginning because he's a very intelligent man which makes it all the worse now that he's gone totally ridiculous, but he didn't pay it much attention. He didn't comment on it at all even though I asked him. It was as if it had nothing to do with him. To me it was obvious that he was making a fool of himself with younger people. I mean they would think,"What's this age-ing grandfather doing here?" but he didn't recognise himself there.

After a time, as I said, he didn't talk about the impotence — and then he began to get secretive. But before he really went off the rails he'd say it wasn't fair to me . . . and where could he go . . . and what could he do? And a friend of ours, a doctor, not our NHS one, suggested that he should go to see Dr Martin Cole. So he did. He went to the clinic in Birmingham and this Martin Cole told him that he wasn't absolutely impotent. My husband told me he put him in this room with the naked women and he got a climax — well, not properly, but nearly, so this is why Martin Cole told him that he wasn't completely impotent. He also said he was to stop taking his epilepsy pills for three months and he wouldn't be impotent at all. I advised him not to stop taking the pills because I would rather him be impotent. I only ever saw it once when he was a young man but it terrified me when he had a mild fit — I thought it was a stroke at the time.

This is why he doesn't think he has been unfaithful — because he hasn't been having proper intercourse since he can't do it. And it was this ridiculous affair of his that brought it all out. He used to go to Manchester and when I came to take his things to the cleaners I've always gone through his pockets — not for any reason but to take them to the cleaners — and I came across these hotel bills for Mr & Mrs — even though he couldn't make love. Then a little later on I came across letters from a number of girls and then this one girl Susie became an infatuation for him. Apparently everyone knew that he was giving her money and taking her out and then my son found out that he was putting her through this modelling course and there was the receipt for the deposit on her new car. I didn't mind the girl so much. After all he's always had women, men do, don't they? It was our life I was concerned about and what was happening to him in all the other ways as well. She was nothing really — so stupid. She was an ignoramus. And finally I had her round at the house. He was in the room all the time and just didn't say anything and she kept saying to him, "Why don't you speak up?" She agreed they had been on holiday together and, still while he was there, I said, "Did he make love to you?" and she said, "Well, he tried. Because he would want something for his money wouldn't he?" Well, I've learned since that you can be impotent but still turned on by certain things or something. He may have tried it with her like he did with me once or twice, but he never tries it now because of the fear of failing. I'm pretty sure he doesn't have intercourse with her now, although he must have tried but not the full thing. I'm sure he has tried because I look at his trousers because I'm meticulously clean and I always brush every thing and he knows. There has been lipstick on his trousers. He said it was impossible but I'm sure and, on an odd occasion, sperm as well, so he must have tried. Of course he's caught because he doesn't want to admit he's been having intercourse because of the guilt yet he would like to boast just to feel that he is good and virile again. But it can't go on like this. The girl is one thing but his whole way of life is another. He can't continue dressing like that for one thing. It's ridiculous. You can see exactly what kind of man he is by the way he looks now.

   If I had been twenty years younger I would have left him, but after forty years . . . it's such a long time — a long, long time and you can't believe the changes. You can't believe it . . . get it into your head. And you can't just uproot and . . . As it is now I would say that I have become frigid, impotent. I have no cause to be otherwise. The other night he kissed me almost sexually. It was the first time for years and I told him so. I think he must have felt a flood of warmth. I certainly did. Even that was as good as having intercourse to me because it was . . . you know . . . loving. So I suppose it's that I miss more than anything — the warm togetherness that we used to have. Perhaps it will come back . . . or maybe I expect too much.

Here again, the situation is no longer as it was when we talked to the wife. During the intervening months events have proved that she was indeed 'expecting too much'. The man has now left and set up another establishment with the young woman. The last time the wife spoke with us, she seemed to be trying to give herself sufficient nervous energy to contemplate divorce action in the near future.

   Our next contributor presents the story from the point of view of the daughter of a victim. She is a fully qualified doctor of medicine and is regularly attending a 'women's group' where part of her self-appointed agenda of therapy is to come to terms with what happened to her father, and its effect upon her.

The major changes that I notice in my father occurred over the years when I was 13 to 19 — when he was a few years under and over 40 — and they were remarkable on two counts. The changes themselves were very noticeable, that was the first thing; and the second was that they contradicted themselves — and I found that bewildering too.

It began just after my sister had gone to boarding school. Before that my father had never been very affectionate towards me — there had never been any affectionate physical contact. Then, all of a sudden, he began to come into my bedroom at night and sit with me and hug me. It was very unusual and lasted for well over six months. It wasn't sexual in any way, very tame in fact, but I found it too strange to tell anyone about.

During that period he took me away for a weekend or two camping and that was again something new. It was really nice and I enjoyed it, but I was shy about telling even my friends because it was all so unusual . . . and strange. I'm sure my father's weird psycholoigcal attitude — sort of reaching out for something but he didn't know what — had a lot to do with why I felt uncomfortable.

After a year or so of this undercurrent of strangeness I began to notice that he was drinking a lot more. Up to that time he'd been a social drinker in the main. At times he would get drunk but before he would always get incredibly polite when he had had too much. My mother and I thought it was funny and quite sweet. But now it was different. There was one night in particular that I remember; late at night I heard the car and when he didn't come in for a long time I went outside to see what was happening. He was lying on the grass flat out. At the time I thought he was sick or dead and I panicked and ran for mother. She soon appeared to have things under control and said, "He's OK don't worry about it." But after that he began to drink more every time he went out — and he also went out much more, spending really quite a lot of time away from home. And now when he got drunk, instead of being nice as he used to be, he became very nasty and hurtful to be with.

Allied with this change of drinking pattern was his sudden switching of friends. He cut himself off from all his old friends and surrounded himself with a host of younger men who didn't demand anything of him. He seemed to like the idea of being with all these young men. He would just sit quietly with them, completely silent, and enjoy the camaraderie. That's what he called it, but it was all very superficial. It had a bad effect on my mother too. Not only did she disapprove of the drinking but she missed their old friends very badly. And just to make things worse for her — and for my father as well I suppose — she had a hysterectomy around this time. It was depressing and confusing for me because I couldn't understand it. I couldn't see that there was anything to get to grips with although I knew something very strange was happening.

The second major change came about towards the end of that period, when I was 18 to 19. I had decided that I wanted to do medicine and he didn't want me to. He resisted it very strongly and wouldn't support me at all — never. Most of the time he would make angry scenes about it. There was only one occasion when he was nice. That was when I failed my exams one year. I suppose he thought that would make me pack it in and when I didn't all the old nastiness came out again. I'm sure that the reasons were that he was annoyed because I had had the audacity to try in the first place, and irritated that I'd been able to do something he had wanted to do. He had trained in medicine himself but had failed and had opted out. His father had wanted him to go into medicine so, when his father died, I think he was overcome by guilt and tried but couldn't make it. This was his way of revenging himself on me for making him appear inadequate I suppose, because he used to put me down in front of my friends and old family friends in ways that would absolutely floor them. In fact, some of them dropped him completely — but some stuck to him. At this time the antagonism was really bad: for no reason at all he would call me a slut although he wasn't accusing me of sluttish conduct. It was as if all the venom and resentment he felt about life and his work were directed at me.

Actually, he was successful at his job — credit manager with an international group — until he was about 40. Previously he had been getting regular promotion and very good money but then he started to run downhill. He seemed to lose interest. He was still quite diligent but he lost the spark he used to have. He said he wouldn't get any further unless he immersed himself in company politics and that wasn't his scene.

He became very nervy and depressed. Then he got funny obsessions. At one time he got a thing on skin cancer. Before, he used to love the beach and being in the sun but after, when we went on the beach he'd wear almost full dress and sit under the beach umbrella and never go swimming. At about the same time he suddenly became very concerned about getting thin — which didn't suit him at all. He just started to eat dramatically less. He wouldn't go on a proper diet or a carrot juice fad because then he could be pinned down about what he was doing, whereas if he was just eating less he could say he wasn't very hungry and no-one could get at him for that. It also came out in his clothes. At times he would wear the most outlandish things and then at others he would get very elegant and spend a lot of time looking at himself in mirrors. Sometimes he looked absolutely ridiculous. Although he looked fairly young still, he had lost his looks — but he didn't think so. At times, he even thought he was as fit and healthy — and good-looking — as he was in his youth . . . but of course it wasn't true. He'd seldom come out in the open about what he was doing, or thinking, or feeling. He started to say things in such a way that if you took it up with him he could deny saying it or meaning it. He was difficult to pin down. He didn't like that at all, so it was impossible to have a logical, rational discussion with him. Even now, our conversations are not easy. He's out of the 'work' trouble because he switched to farming and he seems to be making that work. If we ever manage to sit down together and start to talk at all it's about his problems on the farm — and then he can talk for hours on end. I suppose it's therapeutic for him — but he doesn't want to know about me. Firstly he was threatened by me doing medicine. Now he's threatened because I've passed that up for a time. He objects to me being qualified but not working as he thinks I should. He envied my success and now he envies what he calls my failure — but it's really what he wanted to do himself. He always really resented me being dependent upon him when I was young — having to do a job he didn't like to support a family — not unreasonably I feel , , , even if that's the way our culture works it still probably doesn't feel very good. He can't come to terms with the fact that I take a job for a time and, when I don't need or don't want to, I don't work, and his criticisms all stem from him wanting to do precisely that.

I'm sure that my father thinks his relationship with my elder sister is better than the one he has with me. She's married and settled in Australia with two children and doesn't have a career or anti-establishment thoughts of any kind. But that also goes back a long time to the beginning of the menopause thing because my mother said of his behaviour at the time, "Your father really fell in love with your sister," and I suppose that is what he would have done with me when he started to hug and kiss me — that is, if I had responded properly.

Even so, every so often, there are sparks of something really nice about him. But in general he hasn't got over what happened at 40 or so. He's stayed very cold and close and it's almost impossible to get through that wall of his — and there's no way that you can get him to talk about himself. He'll talk about the farm, but what he feels about himself is something he keeps for himself alone now. It doesn't seem to be very optimistic to me and I know my mother has given up hope.

Janet R. . . . . . is the wife of John whose case is covered on p.93 in his own words. Here Janet tells what she feels like from the position of wife and intimate, involved observer of what she herself defines categorically as the male menopause.

I remember my father going through a very difficult time around the menopause. He used to fall over a lot. He never hurt himself but he got very depressed and would cry a lot. He would just sit and cry. He was in his late forties and I was courting. My mother used to say that he didn't want to lose me. He said "I shan't live to see you married."

For a year or two around that time he thought he had a tumour on the brain. He hadn't of course; it was all in his imagination, all in his mind . . . all to do with him getting a very bad case of the male menopause.

I can remember it all very clearly now. I used to laugh when my mother or anyone else used to refer to men having the male menopause because they don't have physical changes like women. But now I don't laugh any more. It's tragic.

But it hasn't taken John in the same way as it did my father. With John it's much more a case of looking for his youth again. You see, one of the problems of having your children young and close together is that you are still young when they no longer need you. If we had waited a few years, or planned them over a longer distance, he would have got over this time of life before feeling the children no longer needed him to support them. It really does seem to me that he is just seeking for his youth again — and especially by looking for younger women.

He's always liked women ever since I've known him, but I didn't realise until earlier this year when he began this association with the woman he's now involved with . . . I didn't realise he needed it to give him back what he thought he was losing. I did know earlier that something was wrong but I put it down to his overworking. I mean, anything that John does he puts his heart and soul into and he was coming home later and later every night and getting tired and irritable — and un-interested in us as a family. At that time there were two of the children still at home, the last one having left only recently.

At that time I kept on and on at him, that if he didn't ease up on his work he was going to have a breakdown. I could see him heading this way. But he kept saying that the work had to be done and there was nobody else to do it . . . so he had to. However, he did admit that he was irritable and showing signs of strain. Now I know that it was a combination of that overwork   and the guilt he felt about starting with the other woman. But it wasn't until later that it became clear to me that another woman was involved.

In the end I just had to tackle him about the terrible build-up of stress that had been going on. It was prompted by his getting very, very angry with me. He would go for a whole day without speaking — or if he did, he would be snappy. It came to a head one Sunday afternoon when we went for a walk. He was in one of his moods and wouldn't let me hold his arm. It was that more than anything that made me wonder if there was another woman. I said to him that evening, "What's wrong?" and he said that communication between us wasn't very good, and that it was just him and that he was tired. I got impatient and just said right out, "Look; is there another woman?" and he said, "Yes."

I was shattered. But the minute he told me there was another woman I knew who it was because he had brought her home a few times. I had met her in my own home! So, as soon as he'd said it, I knew. I said, "Who is it?" and he said, "Does it matter?" I said I wanted to know and he told me it was R. .

After that, it all sort of drifted on. I was upset that night — tired and shattered — but we talked about it for a long time. I don't think either of us got any sleep. We just talked and talked.

The next day I was in an awful state but then things began to get a little better and we drifted on. Then this post at L. . . . came up and John said he wanted us to make a fresh start and that coming to L. . . . would give us the opportunity to do that. He said he would break off with the other woman. They would have a whole day together and that would be their farewell. And he did that; took her out and then he said that was to be the break. We were to move up to L. . . . and review the situation at the end of a year. I believed him.

About four or five days before we were due to leave I said, "Look, I want you to be absolutely honest with me. Do you want me with you in L. . . .? I don't want to get up there for you to tell me that you don't want me." He said, "No, I genuinely want you in L. . . . and I want to make a fresh start." That was months ago of course, and in fact he's never given her up. When we moved up here he phoned her every night. It seems that she was quite prepared to give John up and I respect her for that, but John's been doing all the chasing. She had no way to get in touch with him easily, so it had to be him — he's always after her although she was prepared to make the break.

But the fault's not all on John's side by any means. I can't pretend that I've got no faults and that I'm not to blame for the way the situation has developed over the years. Of course, it's easier to see this when you're looking back — but not at the time. I must confess that I've neglected him and I haven't been as careful . . . I haven't given him the attention that I should have, the attention that he obviously needed.

I made a big mistake in not letting on what I really felt. You see, I was brought up in a home where my parents rowed quite a bit and they rowed quite openly. I always said as a child I would never row with my husband and I've never done so. Even now we've not had a real row, and I think this was wrong. I would even lie to John when he asked me if I was upset. I would say, "No" and be seething inside but not admit it. I've learned about that and I don't think it's too late to change — but John does.

Anyway, I suppose there must be many couples like that. That's not enough to make the male menopause so bad. There were other things that disturbed him as much if not more — although he may not admit it. For example, he did say once, not so long ago, that he was frightened of getting old. It quite shocked me. It was to someone else outside the home. Someone asked him a direct question and said, "Are you afraid of getting old?" and he said, "Yes, I am very frightened." It shocked me because both of us have had a very strong religious belief and I'm not afraid of dying. But I didn't think that John was worried about getting old and what came with it . . . and death. But then he's lost all his religious faith. He still has the belief in God but he doesn't want anything to do with God. I myself am still strongly religious. I've tried to talk to him about our faith as well as us trying again but every time I try he is so verbally nasty that I've had to give up.

He's changed in so many ways that although I'm being more honest about my feelings it doesn't make any difference to him. He's taken to growing a beard which I think is significant. He's only just done that and he knows it is something that I hate and loathe in men. Over the years we've always laughed about it because beards are a 'thing' with me. I just can't bear beards. Men who grow beards always seem to me to be a bit effeminate. I think it's a kind of virility status symbol. I don't think John has done it deliberately to annoy me. It may be to compensate for going bald; it may be because R. . likes him with it; or it may be a final act of defiance against losing his youth. It's ridiculous really, because it makes him look older. But of course the other girl did tell him that it made him look younger.

Then he got so that he wanted to be slim — and he has lost a lot of weight. So I stopped giving him potatoes and got dry biscuits instead of bread — and we don't have suet puddings like we used to. And actually he does look a lot better from a health point of view as well as appearance. But he's started changing his way of dressing as well. He has bought a lot of new clothes. He said it was because the college didn't like him dressing in jeans and casual things. He needed better clothes to keep up with the professor's requirements . . . or so he said. It's quite a contradiction really because he gave his best suit away before we came up here, and then he said. "They don't like me to wear casual clothes." In the past he's never been bothered about the way he's dressed — never all that bothered about his appearance. He's not been scruffy, but apart from his trousers that I couldn't get for him, I've always bought his clothes. He's never before been interested in going and buying clothes. So that's a big change.

But more than any of that, what is noticeable and hurtful is his attitude to sex. He hasn't had sex with me for a long time. He tells me that I'm physically distasteful to him. He actually used that word, distasteful, and he said to have sex with me now his feelings would be such that he might as well get into bed with a prostitute. I've asked him if he wouldn't just allow me to express my feelings for him but he refused. And there is nothing I can do about it apart from physically attacking him. But there were times when John was absolutely impotent and I put it down to him being over-tired. We did talk about it, but only superficially. He'd say, "I'm sorry but it's just impossible. I can't manage it." All I could do was to say that it was all right; he was tired; and I understood. I thought it was the stress and strain of work and that it would pass. I suppose that things are different with this girl and that over the years he got tired of me — and bored.

I can't honestly see that it can be anything else except an attempt to cope with his menopause by going to bed with a younger woman and proving that he's still youthful and virile in his own mind. It must be since I don't think there's anything particularly attractive about R. . I can't see any other reason. I mean if she was a gorgeous blonde I could understand it, but I would describe her as very ordinary . . . very ordinary indeed. She even giggles a lot and this spoils her appearance quite a bit. When I've been around conversation has been very difficult between her and me — predictably I suppose. But I do find it difficult to see what her appeal is. So it must be in John's mind — and that's where most of his menopause is too, I'm sure.

The major development in this case since we first met the couple is that John has now left his wife, and is convinced that his condition and his handling of it *has* caused serious problems for his children in their own socio-sexual relationships. He blames himself for the break up in their relationships — one in a marriage and the other in an 'informal engagement' of long standing.

From the point of view of 'outside looking in', we move to a female doctor's opinion that suggests that the coincidence of the wife's menopause and the stresses within a marriage are factors of significance.

Dr Prudence Tunnadine is the Training Secretary of the Institute of Psycho Sexual Medicine. Here she puts forward her own views which are not of course necessarily those of the Institute.

As an emotional entity, the male menopause is a very real thing indeed. It is no respecter of social rank. Indeed I would suggest that it is almost universal amongst men. They strive to create and provide for a family and then suddenly say to themselves, "I've got there . . . and now what?"

As a result of no more than one sexual experience with their wives that is a bit duff they may think they have become impotent. They have been very faithful and the impact of this single experience is sufficient to make them think, "My youth has gone." A lifetime's fidelity can make a man very vulnerable in this way and he needs to be taken very seriously.

Should this stage of development coincide with the wife's menopause it can be doubly trying — since they have just as difficult a time as a woman when trying to come to terms with the fact that their children have grown up. Sparks can fly in all sorts of ways: some start trying to live it up through their children and grandchildren — and that's hopeless.

For others it is a real mental and emotional crisis simply because they haven't thought about middle age — what it might do to them and what they might do about it. Suddenly the house is paid for and the kids have gone — and there is nothing but emptiness. For some men the feelings of futility are tremendously alarming.

Some men wonder whether their children value them at all. Some men feel threatened by their sons. After all, none of us is that confident right the way down to our subconscious and what needs to be recognised is that men have these uncertainties just as much as women. But whereas women are *allowed* to have their uncertainties, men are supposed to be lions — the masters of the jungle. And some of them will respond in role. They will bluster and flail about, taking girl-friends to prove they are still what they were supposed to be.

It's very difficult to know how to help people. Out of the thirty or so women patients I see each week five or six of them are likely to mention worries they have about their husband's potency. Of course those figures are to a certain extent self-selective since I do tend to specialise in that area of medicine. But it is still a very big proportion — and it reflects the high degree of psychosomatic illness that occurs at middle age. There is no doubt in my mind that a lot of illness at this time may have its sources in these stresses. Businessmen are renowned for their ulcers and coronaries and it is my theory that nice, disciplined, civilised people who don't go about screaming and throwing saucepans eventually express their stress by way of physical illness.

This particularly applies to stress within a marriage. We do really need to change some of our views here. It's unrealistic to continue bringing up our children to believe they'll only fall in love once — and should only sleep with one person until they are 94. For child rearing purposes, I believe that marriage should be a permanent relationship provided that the parents are able to live together, more or less amicably. No better method has been found for the children's welfare. But after the children have matured I think people should perhaps be prepared to break up and start another phase of life with a different partner if they can no longer make each other happy. Although I'm a practising Christian, I don't think it is the end of the world if couples decide to part and make a new life for themselves on their own. This is where it is important of course for women to be able to work and support themselves — and in this aspect it it easier for professional women.

I am sure that if we relaxed some of our rigid attitudes there would be less guilt and stress and fewer of the anxieties around the time we are talking of. I believe, too, that people should be persuaded quite strongly that it is OK to admit to their anxieties and talk them over with a skilled professional. But we do need more counsellors. The GP does tend to be the first port of call and he needs a specially open eye for the, "It's not me but my back," syndrome when often there is nothing wrong with the patient's back. Ideally, one needs a whole collection of counselling services rather like a complex of shops. You see, some people don't like being seen walking into the Marriage Guidance Council offices for example — it labels them as someone with a bad marriage. But, if one walked through a doorway leading to all manner of different counselling services, no-one would know where you were going.

Above all, people need to know where to go to get help and, in this, women do have an easier time than men. Women get sympathy over the garden wall perhaps, but what man's going to confess to his personal worries at the Rugger Club? There really is nowhere, virtually, for a man to go to talk about his problems. There are vicars, but few people believe nowadays — and the majority feel they can't, or don't want to go to a vicar. For this reason we shouldn't knock prostitutes. Some of them do a very good job listening to men's problems. And some of them even know what to do when a man cries. There shouldn't be this, 'Big Boys Don't Cry' nonsense. Men should be allowed to feel free to cry just as much as women.

There is a very serious aspect to all this — and that is that we are frantically trying to provide help for people with sexual problems, and there is never enough help to go around. And with regard to the male menopause, the trouble is that it is much easier to help a woman psycho-somatically than a man — generally speaking that is. A woman who is frigid — actually I hate the word — can be taught to explore herself and helped to enjoy the genital part of her body. This approach can work well and we have a lot of success helping women — but we have not yet developed such a shortcut for men. For them it may be more difficult to get rid of problems of impotence, which are so deeply a matter of confidence.

No doubt we would all like someone to wave a magic wand and get rid of our problems — be they sexual or menopausal, male or female, or that newly arisen myth, "Everybody but me is having multiple orgasms" — but there is no magic solution for any of us.

On p.98 Claire and Des Rayner discuss the effect the male menopause had, not only on Des, but also on their relationship. Here, Claire talks about it from the point of view of an "agony column" writer.

Women do write to me and say, "It's just as though he were having the change of life. Do men have a change of life?" Some GP's are also using the phrase 'male menopause'. Some readers write and say, "My doctor said he might be going thorugh the male menopause. Is there such a thing?"

Sometimes they write back and say it wasn't the husband's problem at all in the end, but theirs . . . it was the mirror symptom — just like a wife being profoundly depressed because of a disorder of her husband's and children getting symptoms of the parents' illness. So it must be considered in the family setting, and it certainly exists in that sense — when the man 'catches' it from his partner. And not just psychologically but with a great deal to do with smell. The sexual smell of the female is arousing to the male and when the female hormone is switched off she may well emit a different smell and this could have a kick-back effect on the spouse. I have a feeling that this phenomenon of acute depression that people have labelled the male climacteric is much commoner among men with wives who are having their menopause than among other men.

Apart from the mirror symptom, what I think brings on this mid-life or potency crisis for both men and women has nothing to do with hormonal changes. It is the sudden intimation of mortality. I mean, I know the feeling myself. Every so often I will look at my 16 year old daughter and see the smoothness and bounciness of her and immediately I am aware of the sagginess of me — you can't avoid it. But a lot of women feel guilty because they envy their children their youth, smoothness, and all the rest. Sexual jealousy also comes into it, together with a lot of resentment of their sexual freedom. Also, suddenly they have got all the things you worked so hard to give them, and you don't like it. Now, in a woman that may be bad enough, but in a man it's even more painful because, somehow, he's still out there fighting the battle as it were. Most women are protected in our society . . . and most men are responsible. For a lot of them, having to face the fact that suddenly their kids are outstripping them and they've reached the top of the tree — and there aren't many trees from which you don't start going downwards after the middle 40's. Generally, a man is over the top and he has people coming up behind and he feels bad about it. He feels bad about the sexual aspect too. You've only to watch the way baboons react when the young ones start trying to steal their girls and showing their sexual potency. The middle aged baboons show depressed behaviours. Similarly, a man may feel utterly depressed when his son is no longer a strapping boy. There are now two men: one young and vigorous, the other tired. It's as though a chap has been pushed somewhere along the line into a cul-de-sac and has only just seen it for what it is and is tearing back to get out in time before they put the gates across the end. A lot of women put it this way in their letters. There was one, for example, "Can you help me find my husband? He got up and took his lunch to go to work a few weeks ago and hasn't come back yet." This was a case of a man who had just quit cold. He had always been a good, quiet husband and all the rest of it. It was a very clear story of a man who suddenly saw that "This is the way it is going to be for always," and shot off in the other direction. The woman was totally bewildered and there was a piece right at the end of the letter that was incredibly touching, "I put a message in the paper about the dog because the dog was missing him too."

Then there is the classic other response and I get a lot of letters saying, "I've been working as such and such for so many years and I want to start a business, run a pub, buy a farm," . . . there's a whole list of them . . . "Please tell me how to." That is the really classic male menopause.

Des has definitely had it, there's no doubt. Fortunately I had a bit more information than most wives so I didn't panic about it, that was one good thing. But it was tedious. I used to feel quite guilty at how irritated I got with him. I would sympathise and understand but I still found it damned boring, honestly. He was awfully good about it and didn't fuss too much but he was very depressed and dreary — and of course it was terribly catching.

One of the things that makes it that much worse now is that we are all healthier than we were. Health brings discontentment. The luxury of looking inside your head about "What do I feel?" . . . "What's going on?" is a luxury we're given because we're not hungry. To the average peasant, the idea of the male menopause would be ludicrous. He would be feeling bloody lucky just to get tomorrow's dinner. The biggest change we have had this century is from aspirations to expectations. Once, people aspired. They hoped. They said, "I hope to be well. I hope to get enough to eat." And if they did they were happy and contented. Everything had worked out well for them and it was marvellous — and if it didn't, well, after all, they had only hoped. But now people expect all these things so when they get success in a job or a loving wife, they don't think, "How fortunate I am," they take it for granted. And if they don't get it, their reaction is, "Why me? What have I done not to get my share?" People are demanding more — and it is a shame, because the more you expect, the less you'll ever get.

Claire Rayner's comments provide a happy bridge from the subjective, inner experience to the completely external world of the press. Claire's views as an agony columnist contrast dramatically with those expressed by Marje Proops (see below). There is no doubt in our minds that the attention the media and the press have given to the idea of the male menopause has contributed greatly to individual and collective opinions on the subject. In fact, wherever we have mentioned our book, the first reaction, as we have already said, was that people were either suffering themselves or knew someone who was. The second reaction was to refer to an article or feature in a newspaper or magazine — or to mention the Parkinson television programme. The subject has mushroomed over the months and has gained acceptance as a myth and as a reality, as a joke and as a deadly earnest conversation topic. Starting with Marje Proops the following pieces show something of the way the matter has been treated by journalists.

QUIET, MAN! MENOPAUSE IS STRICTLY FOR THE BIRDS

My greetings telegram to a man friend who last week celebrated his 45th birthday was not received with the warm gratitude I'd expected.

He rang up not to say thank you, but to tell me all about his male menopause.

It was quite unbearable to listen to him going on about his depression, his backache, his sexual disinclinations, his tiredness, his spare tyre, his greying hair and how nobody appreciated him and how his wife took him for granted and how the children no longer respected him.

"I realise," he said, "why women moan about the change of life, now that I'm obviously going through it."

I asked him if he'd started his hot flushes.

"Not yet," he said, actually taking my ribald question seriously.

Since the idea began to get around that men do experience some kind of emotional slump in middle-age, more and more are eagerly jumping on to the menopause bandwagon, claiming that they, like women, are having to endure the symptoms of the change of life.

It is, of course, utter rubbish. What happens to women is a hormonal change and every doctor with whom I have discussed the possibility of a male menopause, in the strict sense of the word, dismisses it as sheer fantasy.

Men, as one doctor pointed out, have not so far been equipped with ovaries. Nor have they, as yet, started to menstruate.

When baby boys are born with the ability to conceive and give birth, he stated — and quite solemnly — then men can look forward to a change of life similar to that which women experience.

What actually happens to men in middle-age is that they suffer from the same sort of emotional problems which beset many middle-aged women.

Like fear of getting old. Like fear of competition from younger and more virile citizens. Like overweight. Like life losing its excitement. Like stale marriages and boredom and thwarted ambitions.

But while women have all these, plus the real hot flushes and the very real physical symptoms of the menopause, with men it's all in the mind.

I am sorry to have to tell my birthday friend and others of his ilk who feel they deserve special sympathy and understanding at this difficult time of their lives that though they might well need our loving kindness, the menopause has nothing to do with what ails them.

The real change is strictly for the birds.

Reporting on Edward Woodward's return to his wife after ending his affaire with actress Michele Dotrice, Shaun Usher wrote in the Daily Mail:

Baffled and hurt, Venetia Woodward thought her husband was bewitched and found 'the male menopause' the only logical explanation.

Certainly middle age is dangerous. Woodward has been too busy (ironically enough, in a stage comedy about marriage on approval) to watch ITV's *The Nearly Man,* but the situation is the same.

In the series, a 45-ish Labour MP meets a young college lecturer whose frank and calculated admiration and total willingness to surrender simply sweeps him off his feet.

Among ordinary people, the hazard is less serious. A balding middle-aged plumber making eyes at a teenaged typist is likely to be laughed back to safety. In any case, he won't have the financial muscle needed for a mistress.

Actors, on the contrary, are paid to work with pretty girls and expected to flatter and flirt with them. They have the confidence that fame and money bring.

Michele, a lovely young woman with a devastatingly open confiding brand of appeal, worked with Woodward in a stage comedy last year, and the unwitting trap — older man's confidante poise, knowledge; girl's appreciation, turning the clock back — was sprung.

Lynda Lee Potter, writing in the same newspaper:

The ever-increasing manifestation of something called the male menopause is possibly a result of a widespread malaise among men, a fear that nothing will ever get better and may even get worse.

The Guardian treated the subject in a different way:

Men, too can suffer from the menopause. Dennis Barker reports.

THE IMPOTENCE OF MAN'S MIDDLE AGE

Men can die from the menopause if they are unlucky. Most just suffer while their wives endure the symptoms of the "change of life."

"I would like to see some research into this, but at present no one seems keen to do it," Mrs Jean Robinson of the Patients' Association said yesterday.

Mrs Robinson disclaims medical knowledge, but has observed some common patterns in men at the time their womenfolk encounter the menopause.

Doctors (who are mostly men) might be more sympathetic to women's menopausal problems if their effect on men were better known, she says, and will take up the subject at a conference called by MIND, the National Association for Mental Health this month.

Impotence is one serious threat for a man married to a woman who finds intercourse painful because of vaginal atrophy or other menopausal symptoms. He starts to worry about his own potency and his home and sex life can gradually decline.

Some men find themselves enmeshed in arguments caused by

menopausal "nerves" or quarrelsomeness. In one case, the barking of a neighbour's dog became so intolerable to a woman that her husband was obliged to take up the subject.

The obsessive careerist, who has pushed hard all his life and expected his wife to understand his problems may find that her supply of sympathy dries up. She now expects sympathy from him, at a time when her husband is likely to be at a plateau of his career.

Some husbands may have to watch their teenage children leave home because of their mother's menopausal behaviour, which they are too young to understand. He may be relieved to see the children go, thus stopping domestic tension, but at the same time feel that he has been forced to betray his children. Resentment against his wife builds up.

Late arrival at work is a sign of a man at risk. If he gets to office or factory persistently late because he has been having, or avoiding, a row with his menopausal wife, or because he has had to make the breakfast and get the children to school, he creates tensions at work. He may get the feeling he is fighting two battles at once.

Any of these characteristics, but perhaps specially the last, could be a warning sign of premature coronary attack, which might be fatal. "I want men to write to us," Mrs Robinson said, "to say how the menopause has affected them. It could be that marriages that break up at this time need not if there were better mental health treatment for the wife."

And back again to the Daily Mail for a full page treatment:

Postscript to a much discussed TV special

THE MALE MENOPAUSE

Colin Reid writing today for Femail

IS IT A MAN'S SUPREME ALIBI?

Was there ever a better slice of Men's Lib propaganda than *The Male Menopause* programme put out by Mike Parkinson on BBC TV this week?

What a marvellous excuse for a whole new way of life for all middle-aged husbands and fathers.

We can get away with murder and blame it all on 'the change.' It's just what we've been looking for all these years. And God bless you, Dr Parkinson!

New order

I don't know about you, but I've already got my next five-year plan laid out — five years of fun, frolics and a new order in the home. There'll be no more of this 'good old steady Dad', pushing him around, pinching his seat, beating him up on the tennis court and golf courses and taking him for granted.

From now on Dad is going to be decidedly unsteady — in and out of the home. And I've already put it about the family that what I want is sympathy and understanding while I'm going through this very difficult period.

Furthermore, if they have any love for me at all, they'll let me win for a change at golf and tennis, otherwise it might worsen my condition.

And then where will they all be? Who'll pay the mortgage? Who'll win the bread? Who'll answer the back door on Saturday mornings?

Oh, yes! With one bound, sir, you too can jump out of your life of humdrum frustration. Join the Magnificent Menopausal Men.

If your wife finds you wining and dining some fabulous dolly from the office typing pool all you do is look wounded and say, 'But it's my emotional hormones, dear — you know how it is when you reach my time of life.

Your life swims before your eyes and you say, "Where am I going? What have I done with myself? What does it all mean?" I must recapture some of my youth, it's the only answer. And please stop threatening me with that bottle.'

Eyes rolling

If we hog the bathroom in the morning there'll be no more pounding on the door. Our families will know that we are engaged in therapeutic matters like looking in the mirror, pulling in our paunches, examining our teeth and talking to ourselves as befits Menopausal Man.

If we complain about our aches and pains we shall get a sympathetic hearing instead of that business of eyes rolling heavenwards and mutters of:

'Oh God, he's at it again — it's indigestion! You eat too much! You drink too much! And isn't it funny you always get a pain when I ask you to mow the lawn?'

We can even lash ourselves up in all the latest gear and fancy hairstyles. The Wrinklies are moving in, youth is stepping aside. We're in for a new life, men — that's if your families saw the TV programme or have carefully digested the reviews.

Wisely, indeed with brilliant sixth sense, I had insisted that we all watch it. They wanted to watch James Garner in *The Rockford Files,* but I put it to them straight: was James Garner more important than their Dad?

Yes, they said. But I beat them to the switch.

Even so, I had to keep shutting them up. 'Be quiet, this is vital information, it concerns your whole future,' I told them as all the male menopausal symptoms were trotted out. 'And stop laughing, will you? It's serious.'

'Male menopause? It's all in the mind,' said my wife.

'Of course it's all in the mind!' I said, 'Are you saying that my mind doesn't matter? Are you only interested in my body?'

You see, already I was getting one of my funny turns. It's part of growing older.

This kind of treatment is not atypical of how the menopausal male tackles his own predicament in social conversation, nor of how he may find others responding to him. As Paul Rimmer points out, many men refer to it in jocular terms, but in reality it is no joke. Some people may refer to it in a facetious mode, but the reality of what is happening will be lurking somewhere in their minds.

This back-to-front paradoxical system of coping with the experience is a personal expression of what the victim thinks and feels and also a considered attempt to communicate some of what is symptomatic of the male menopause. This is what makes it an entity in its own right. It is not just depression or melancholia stemming from ageing, or nostalgia for things, people and times past. It is not just secondary impotence caused by psychological or organic factors or both. It is not just the change of life (or 'the change') and saying 'Goodbye Youth, Hello Death, now I am over the hump'. And it is certainly not the menopause proper. No; the addition of the prefix 'male' takes us straightaway into a topsy-turvy world of bizarre values. The essence of the male menopause lies in its self-contained contradictions. It is, in its classic sense, truly redolent of the *absurdity of the human condition*.

The menopausal male, who although he will always blame other people and 'things', sets himself up as his own Aunt Sally in a ridiculous fairground for the middle-aged. Such self-destructive behaviour patterns really deserve nothing but contempt, but since the victims disclose a gross sense of failure, inadequacy and vague but furious impotence, they command nothing but compassion, sympathy and understanding — for a time. In any case, such feelings are wasted on the menopausal male who is quite unable to accept, accommodate or exploit any of them to good purpose — such is the extremity of his self-defeating posture.

3 From the inside...looking out

I'm sure men get it just as much as women — without the obvious
physical symptoms I mean, well not all of them any way — just
psychologically. What happens is that you get to 45-46 and you say,
'That's it I suppose . . . there's not much left now . . . it's all over . . .
finished and done.' I've thought about it a lot and I'm sure it will happen
to me. I haven't brooded on it, but I know it's on the way . . . and I'm
only 28. Oh yes; the male menopause will get you. That's for sure.

Unsolicited comment from a visiting carpenter who happened to glance
at the manuscript.

Our visitor may not have been totally right, but we have come across
only a handful of people out of the hundreds we have talked to who
actually reject the idea of the male menopause. For many of them it
means the same thing: depression and impotence; but there are others
who see it in all kinds of lights. This in itself is part of what the male
menopause is all about. The victim sees things in different and usually
strange ways. As Kant says, "We see things, not as they are, but as we
are." And what has struck us most forcibly while researching the
subject has been that if a man feels he has the male menopause, the
chances are that he has — in the terms we are now using to describe
the syndrome.

We have already outlined (on p.22) the broad spectrum that
contains most of the responses to an onslaught of the condition: going
with the symptoms; ignoring them; over-responding to them; and
exploiting them — for good or ill. For example, some men use the idea
as an excuse for chasing girls, while others use it as an excuse to avoid
the challenges of sex altogether. These latter opt out of sexual relationships completely — even with their wives. Running away from sexual
'threats', they can leave their wives to many years of deprivation of
sexual activity. This is one of the reasons why Robert Chartham has got

angry in the past: he has experienced too many cases where a husband has callously allowed his wife to suffer as a result of his cowardly retreat under cover of what is for him perhaps a total misuse of the phrase.

Some men read the symptoms as heralds of maturity welcoming what they think will be a period of long sought after calm. Others read them as harbingers of senility, a condition they have no wish to embrace. For some men it is just a feeling process and for others it is a set of near reflex actions. They are quite unaware of what is happening to them or how they are responding; the dramatic changes in their behaviour ("I don't know what has come over him") go unnoticed by the victims themselves. However, for most men it is a period of considerable thought and they get involved in heavy introspection. Since many are also more than articulate we can now have the benefit of their comments straight from the experiential level. Here then is another personal testimony from a sufferer.

John R. . . . . . is currently improving his academic qualifications by attending a full time degree course related to his career in social work. He is 46 and after leaving school joined the Navy. He started a second profession in the probation service and later in more general social work. He married his wife Janet twenty three years ago. They are the same age and have three adult children. John and Janet were both religious for many years. She still is; he is not, and this is merely one way in which his 'questioning' of life and his place in it has alienated him from her and much of his past.

The incident which threw his conflicts into the open occurred about five years ago. John attended a group training course that was non-hierarchical in everything but personal qualities. For once John R. . . . . . was on show as a man and not a professional symbol or cipher. He welcomed the change, having formed the impression that he was only respected or appreciated (if at all) because of his position as a lecturer in a college that trains social workers. He was flattered when the training group democratically elected him as 'leader'. He was reassured that, as a person, he had some sort of presence and purpose.

He was completely thrown, however, when a young woman on the course made overt sexual advances to him. He found it disturbing, disconcerting, exciting and guilt provoking — and was completely unable to handle it. Although immensely flattered he resisted the temptation to sleep with her — but it started him on the road to reappraisal.

The course put him into a state of euphoria for several weeks but Janet was unable to share it because she couldn't understand it. This brought about strong feelings of resentment from John and slowly he descended into a pit of despair and depression that he later realised had been opening up for years. Talking about this 'rock-bottom depression' John said, "It was inevitable, I suppose, that the answer would lie in another woman. Later I met R. . at college and I fell in love with her, but if it hadn't been her it would have been somebody else."

This is how John sees what he calls the climacteric. His wife's assessment of the situation (she doesn't pull any punches and calls it the male menopause, for which John criticises her) can be found on p. 76.

The first signs were by no means dramatic: I noticed an occasional shortness of breath and became aware of the old bald head. Once I was sitting in the barber's chair and previously he'd always thinned it out on the top. This time he said, "Are you sure you want it thinned out?" — little things like that.

The major realisation came out of the blue as it were. I was driving to work one day and I suddenly thought, "If I were to get killed, who would care?" And I decided that no-one would. My wife had her nursing career and her religion — she would just immerse herself in those. My children were all grown up and although they might grieve and be sad for a time, they would get over it and recover without a problem. Then there were my students. Well; they would be sorry I think, but there's always someone to replace you — nobody's indispensable. It was a terrible feeling. All in all, it was like being in the middle of a rock-bottom depression with no way up or out.

It brought me face to face with my life in a new way. I remember saying to myself, "Well then John, what's for real about this world? Just take a look at yourself. You can almost plot out the sort of behaviour that is predictable from a middle-aged man going through this and that crisis. You're doing exactly that. What are you? Are you a puppet — and someone pulls the strings — or are you a human being with responsibility for what you are doing and what's going on? What's real about your life? What's real about you?"

I remember thinking that I was like somebody going on to the stage with one pre-set role all set out, and that I was just going through it piece by piece. I asked myself if I was being myself and if I was making my own decisions. Was any of it real? Or was I just a sort of performing observer of my own life? The questions were really 'ouchy' and I felt the crunch had come.

I reviewed what I felt about life, people, things — and above all, me. And I discovered that all I had had for some time was a sense of depression and dissatisfaction with life generally. A sense of kicking against the pricks. A sense of questioning one's virility — and one's sexual attractiveness.

I was flailing about in total ignorance of what was going on, because, although I'd noticed a few articles in newspapers and magazines, there is very little worthwhile stuff that has been written. It's one of those taboo areas that's not aired or talked about a lot. My wife tends to see what I'm doing as only to be expected of a man of my age — and that's a real put-down in a sense. You see, I've always referred to what's happening to me as the 'climacteric', but she calls it the 'male menopause' — and I find that a female chauvinistic thing to do. But I suppose she can't be expected not to be jaundiced about the things I'm doing to try to get out of it all.

For example, there's the sense of attempting something new. The need to prove oneself in several new spheres all at once. The fact of seeking out other women — testing out your virility. I mean, even with this relationship I've got with this girl, am I testing out what kind of virile man I still am, or is it something that has more reality and value than that? There's no doubt that I am searching for symbols and status in all kinds of ways, not just to do with virility.

This course I'm taking in L. . . . is a good example. Why should I throw up a fairly comfortable life in P. . . . . to come here and get a qualification that doesn't do a thing for me financially? That is simply because I have no academic qualification and I'm very aware of it. I'm very conscious of the fact that my Principal talks about when she was at Cambridge, and she puts on her hat and gown — and I just sit there in my suit. In the educational world your academic qualifications are what count. They are the things that give you your status. It's a status thing. I'm really conscious of not having the status.

Everybody says, "Oh, you don't need an academic qualification. It's your merits we're worried about. You're a good lecturer," and all this kind of thing. But when it comes down to brass tacks as well as the really symbolic instances, you very clearly are low down on the status situation.

I suppose it didn't matter so much a few years ago when I was in the probation service still, because I was professionally qualified and academic qualifications didn't matter. But, on this course, I knew I was sticking my neck out. I'm next to the oldest — I thought I was going to be the Daddy but I'm not — and I'm competing against bright young things who have their degrees, their years in university, and their years of field work behind them. They are intellectually much brighter than me and they have the ability to retain things which I don't have. The old grey cells, you know. I find it pretty difficult and I have to work extremely hard to keep up. I'm really sticking my neck out on this lot.

I hope, of course, that it will be an advantage to me in getting other jobs, but I'm very happy in social work at the moment. However, my old Head of Department thought it advantageous to be able to put my name on the list of tutors with a good academic qualification because he's hoping to expand the course. It's the politics of higher education. He's hoping to impress the CNAA, the Academic Council and the Council for Educational Training by saying, "We've got this tutor with blah, blah, blah, etc." It just means to me personally that I can say that I've got an academic degree which I didn't have before. It's the status thing again. I was accepted for two courses and the other was much more suited to my educational needs and I evaluated it as a much better course — but it just did not have the academic qualification. I suppose I must accept that most of it comes back to the idea of testing and proving one's virility again, but in all kinds of ways and that must be behind the climacteric crisis.

I'm not well acquainted with the basic theories of the stages of human development, but there must be stages and each of them presents its own kind of crisis. For men, I see the male menopause as a crisis that for one reason or another they either work through or produce some sort of positive or negative response to. You get examples of these cases in the papers every day. Last Sunday there was this case of a man who had a family and was a director of a firm who is now registered alongside his son at University. He is taking the same degree and is going to give up his directorship and teach in a foreign country. Well, that's his response to the crisis. He's working his way through it and it looks as if he and his wife have been able to work through it together — both of them.

It might well be that if this girl and I hadn't become involved with one another, I might not have woken up to the crisis. I might not have responded either. But I suppose someone else would have woken me up I expect. I was in an awakening process, but she was the catharsis and really put the finger on things as far as I'm concerned. If she hadn't done I may well have stagnated, which is a lot of people's response to the crisis situation. You get sort of stagnant relationships — I can see it in my own family situation — where people get into this pattern of living and get so used to it that the habits are virtually indestructible. But there's no real closeness in the relationships. They just accommodate each other and outwardly everything is OK. They just sort of trog on: that seems to me the majority way of dealing with the male menopause . . . to trog on.

I don't think any man avoids the male menopause. Mind you, it's a very subjective opinion because it's all much more concrete in a woman: the physical changes — the end of fertility — a new era in life. And with a man you don't get the same sort of physical symptoms. Just as with a woman you can't say the timing is always the same — it doesn't definitely appear between 40 and 45 — the same with a man. It may be 50 to 55 — and, equally important, there are other developmental bits that you get, repeating patterns of earlier events.

Undoubtedly there is a bit of childhood development going on in me now. I'm only just learning how to express aggression properly. Now if you accept a Kleinian model of development then this is going right back to the nine-month-old stage. But I find it very difficult to express aggression, especially to women. I suppose it's the fantasy of omnipotence — that I might really destroy them. Anyway, the relationship I have with R. . is certainly helping me through that stage of development. But they're different for different people.

It's a period of life which is to a greater or lesser extent a crisis time coinciding with major changes in the family situation. I'm currently involved with a man of 42 who has just got married. Now I can't see him going through the same stressful situation. He won't get the male menopause in a bad way because he doesn't have any children that have 'flown the coop'. That's the very bad bit. He's just setting up his relationship with his wife. He hasn't got one that has existed for 23 years. He's never been married at all. In fact, he's been a 'mummy's boy'. For me it's related to family life and the change. Before there has been the emphasis on the bringing up of the children, the providing of the home and all that goes with the nest syndrome. Suddenly, this is a function that ceases and there has to be a readjustment, a re-focusing and a re-emphasis in the marriage relationship.

It's all to do with catching sight of the end of life: 'Hell, I've only got thirty years left. I'm already half-way there . . . if I manage to get that far." It's all to do with all those things I've wanted to do and haven't been able to do. Before, I've always been able to say, "There are the children. They are the limiting factor." But they're not any longer — and I still can't do them. I see my faculties declining, virility waning. My ability to be able to grasp things, particularly them. OK, if you wanted me to do an essay and you gave me plenty of time to prepare, then I could cope. I could go to books and all that kind of thing. But to do anything off the top is now quite beyond me.

Then again I was listless. I was bored. And I was constantly questioning my sexual attractiveness because I was sexually bored. It's difficult to be entirely objective about it because of course my wife was involved, and I didn't know what she was feeling — but I was very dissatisfied and very bored. Janet had this attitude that the woman's part was a very passive one and for me sexual intercourse is a mutual, joint, together act. As with life, I can't accept that one should be passive and the other active. So I was really looking twice at my sexuality.

A lot of women, especially women students, have felt attracted to me as a person. But I've always seen myself as a 'father figure' rather than a man in my own right and that's a real difference. Only the other day a kid I met in one of the drug therapy units said, "I bet you would make a smashing Dad." And that's how I've seemed to be . . . to me that is . . . paternal, not a sexually attractive man. So when this young woman, R. ., made it clear that she saw me in that kind of light I was not just surprised, I was flattered and it made me weak — but there was also the guilt because in my morality at that stage, it was just verboten. So it was not without its conflicts.

Nor is the future clear and certain. Intellectually I can see only one clear path, but coming to terms with it emotionally is a different matter. For example, there's my mother, goodness knows what she's going to say when I have to tell her that I want to separate from Janet. My fantasies of aggression and destruction come up again quite hideously. My fear is that it might kill her even. She's very frail, about 80, and she has such strong views about divorce and expresses them so fully that I'm quite frightened to tell her — but I suppose I shall have to at some stage.

When I think about it quietly I know that if I were to stay with Janet and retain the same pattern of life, within two or three years I'd be in such a state of depression that I'd probably stick my head in the oven. Well, I don't know if I would really, but that would be the sort of depth that I could get to. I would be totally frustrated and certainly not functioning at work, and probably kicking her like hell all the time and really making her life utterly miserable. So it does seem a pretty clear decision there. All I have to do is to put it into action.

As far as the future is concerned with R. ., well, there is no under-standing about this and it is very much a matter of hope on my part, but I hope that she will feel that she would like to share life with me. And that brings up more ambivalent feelings because she wants children. To my mind she is a very maternal person and would be a good mother but whether at my age I'd be able to cope with having kids around the house and live with having my nose put out of joint by the attention she would give to them — attention that I would want — I just don't know.

Then again, in fifteen years I'll be coming up for retirement and she'll still be in her prime. That is another thought that frightens me. But on the other hand I've had twelve months experience of the sort of relationship that I never dreamed existed. That may sound a bit fairy tale, but it's true. It's been an open sort of relationship which I'd never come across before. An openness to express the negative as well as the positive. R. . has thumped me at times, physically, but it's all right — it really is all right. It took me a bit of understanding — but it really is all right. Now, Janet could never do that. She couldn't even tell me when she was upset with me. And of course R. . can make me feel on top of the world which Janet isn't able to do.

Really, I shall have to leave Janet regardless of R. . as a matter of personal survival. That's absolutely necessary, and fortunately for me, because it's very important, the children are not actually against it. That helps relieve the pressure that comes from feeling responsible for Janet while she finishes this special course of further nursing training. It may be stupid, but I feel I ought to try to maintain a certain standard so we're living together through all this. I don't think the children understand it really. I don't see how they can but they think of Janet and I as being reasonable people, who don't do things without there being some good reason, so they've just gone along with it. Its made them re-evaluate their own relationships and look at marriage all over again. So my crisis is theirs too I suppose.

We've already heard from Claire Rayner herself (p.82) but here she is in the dual role of wife and adviser, talking with her husband, Des, about the impact that the male menopause had on him and their relationship:

DES: People usually stick at 35 or 40. In my case I chose 37. I suddenly felt that being over 35 with 40 well on its way was time to think, "Where do I go from here?" Generally, one thinks of a man at around 37 as having a nice established career, being set in his ways and all the rest of it. But it wasn't like that for me. I'd tried all sorts of things: I'd been in the theatre; I'd been in the forces; I'd done advertising and I was back in it and hating it; I still wanted to write and wasn't being very successful; and I thought about painting, but not terribly seriously since I'd always painted. A whole conglomeration of things came together, and were sparked off by a birthday.

We have always gone out on each others' birthdays — a dinner and a show — but when Claire said to me "Where are we going?", I said, "We're not." I have an October birthday — the 31st, Hallowe'en — which can account for a lot, and we just sat on either side of the fire and looked at each other.

CLAIRE: You didn't. You looked into the flames . . . and you glowered.

DES: Oh yes, she said, "What are you looking at?", and I said, "My lost youth going up the chimney."

CLAIRE: It wasn't quite as dramatic as that immediately. But that was the theme. That was the starting point of the acute depressions.

DES: It's only recently begun to be accepted that men do go through something. Generally, women's symptoms are more obvious; they can be seen to be happening and are therefore more acceptable — just because they occur in the body. But I am convinced that what goes on in a man's mind is just as important. I'm not saying that a woman's physical changes are not accompanied by things going on in her mind but merely that there is the one to substantiate the other — and with a man you haven't.

CLAIRE: It may well be worse for men, for those who know there is no physical, physiological change. Women are allowed their miseries and headaches, their blues and depressions. They have their label — an actual physical thing that you can see.

DES: And there is still this thing — OK, a woman goes through menopause, gets depressed and sheds a few tears and all the rest of it, but if a man sheds a few tears it's, "Oh, that's not done, old boy," And the usual remedy from the medical profession is to hand out the pills, and I got all that. I had anti-depressants, sleeping pills and tranquillisers. All of them I had — and there is a terrible trap attached to them which I wasn't warned about: they contribute to impotence. There was I saying, "Who am I? What am I? Where am I? etcetera, etcetera . ." and I couldn't even get it up. I couldn't even have that pleasure.

CLAIRE: There's a real Catch 22 situation here. If a doctor says to a patient, "I'm giving you these tablets but don't be worried if they put you off your oats because that might happen," it's going to cause it to happen. If the doctor doesn't tell the patient and it happens — then he should have done. Either way he is in the wrong.

DES: There were other side effects to all the tablets — not the least of which was the doziness. I remember I was on the phone once and I could hear this voice way in the distance saying, "Desmond, Desmond, are you there?" I had just momentarily gone off. It happened again a few days later at an office conference. I could feel myself going off again and there was this voice in the distance saying, "Can we have your opinion on this layout? Desmond what do you think of this layout? Wake up!" It was a spiral and I felt terrible.

About the time of the third depression I was working at home, and that was a bit traumatic as well, writing and painting. It was Whitsun and we went to friends — a very hot day. On the way home I remember saying to Claire, "What happened at such and such a time? The day's gone and I can't remember it going." Claire said I had some tablets in the morning and slept all day.

CLAIRE: Of course, we told good friends about it. In fact, one of them actually rushed off himself to Devon dairy farming and we're worried about him too because there is no question that that was menopausal.

DES: It's a restlessness — a wanting something different — and probably my saving grace was that I was able to give up what I had been doing for 12 years and change my way of life.

CLAIRE: Even then it was frightening and probably made more acute by that change because the first few months were very, very difficult.

DES: It's beginning to pay off now, but it did take two years . . . which I suppose in some respects isn't too bad. Anyway, to get back to this Whitsun. I got home and I suddenly realised that my problems and my worries — the causes of my depression — weren't coming from within me. They were outside circumstances, essentially.

CLAIRE: There were outside circumstances as *well.*

DES: It was the thing of my work not being accepted, not being loved — that sort of feeling. Everything I wrote had to be accepted; everything

I painted had to be bought.

CLAIRE: Which is not exactly realistic.

DES: And I realised this and I thought, "Sod this, I'm not taking any more tablets," and I emptied them down the loo — and I haven't taken any since.

I was in fact on and off them all those years from 37 to 43 — more off than on in all honesty I suppose — but it happened this way: they affected my potency *very much.*

CLAIRE: And we noticed!

DES: But the tablets didn't affect me that way until after a few months.

CLAIRE: But he wouldn't believe me. I said not to worry, it's only the pills, it doesn't matter.

DES: I was thinking in terms of the age thing, "Right, well, this is it!"

CLAIRE: He still wouldn't believe me in spite of all the reassurance I could give him. You see, I wasn't anyone who *knew* about these things; I was the woman he slept with. Why should I know?

DES: I think in some ways it was worse being married to Claire who was answering everybody's problems. I think I expected her to say, "There, there dear; if you do this, this and this it will be all right."

CLAIRE: Which is what all the readers want as well and I have said it a million times, "I've never solved anyone's problem in my life." What I've ever done, hopefully, is to point people in the direction of solving their own, or provided them with information, or a wet shoulder. That's all I'm for. There is no short answer, but this time he wanted a miracle.

DES: Sure! Everyone who is unwell in some way or other wants a miracle.

CLAIRE: I spend an enormous amount of time telling people who write letters, "There is no short cut, no magic wand. All a nose operation will change is your nose. It will not change your life."

DES: Fortunately, in our particular circumstances we are probably more vocal than most couples, so we can talk it out.

CLAIRE: But you didn't always believe what I said.

DES: No, but at the time you don't necessarily want an answer. You want a sounding board. You just stand there and let it come back at you. On one occasion I went to see my doctor for something quite different and I started jabbering on and on and I finally said, "I've really come to talk about myself, haven't I?" And he said, "Any time you want to come in for a chat, please do."

CLAIRE: And this is not common. I wish it were because talk is so important. We have a thing in our family which is almost a joke: it was started by my sister-in-law and when everyone is sitting around talking, if you feel the need to tell it out loud, you say MY TURN — ME NOW!

DES: Right! But to compare the male menopause with the female menopause, with a woman it coincides with the time when she feels the family has grown away from her; but with a man it also coincides with the fact that they've been at a job for a certain amount of time — for me twelve years — and he thinks, "Right! Where do I go from here?" So, you're president — what's your next job?

I know that a lot of sociologists are saying that it is not a bad thing to change course in mid-stream. It opens up your horizons. Gives you new interests and goals.

CLAIRE: There are people who go off and open little shops in remote villages and it's great if they can make a go of it.

DES: But a lot of people can't just say, "I'm going to do it," and do it. It isn't as simple as that. With a lot of people it all goes on in their heads.

Oddly enough I'm just working on a play that deals with this aspect — although it's female centred. It's called "The Ubiquitous Mrs Smith". She is a female Walter Mitty, driven into the situation because she's put all her life into her kids, her husband and her home. She's very well educated and just over 40. Her daughter is now going out and about and her husband is well established and there she is at home. What the hell is she going to do? She wants to be a person again so she fantasises into all these situations — and in between manages to have some conversations with her husband in which she says, "I've worked for you. I've worked for the home. I've done all that — and I've got my problems."

Now, I'm going to be very male chauvinistic about this: as I said before, when the woman is going through it, hers is in evidence — she's got an excuse. But if she isn't terribly understanding and knowledgeable about it she'll probably think about the man that he is *opting out* of her problem — instead of him actually *opting in.* It's a very common Catch 22 problem if they have it going together.

Of course, the woman's is more limited by a time factor. It starts at a certain time and lasts for two to three years, and once the hot flushes and everything are over she's had time to accept that her body is not the same as it was — and that's the end of it. But with a man it's a stopping and starting thing and the only approach they can use is the MY TURN — ME NOW idea.

I suppose in many ways it does appear to be much more unrealistic for a man because it's so much more faltering and you can't say, "Look, this is happening to me," because you can't show it — except in the obvious form of impotence.

It certainly wasn't much fun for Claire. I just sort of retreated and sat in a corner as it were. I completely . . . shut off.

We have already quoted cases where the 'young woman thing' seemed the most important fact and many men get hooked on a (renewed?)

search for La Dolce Vita or a Swinging Trip. For some of them the outlet comes in another Hall of Mirrors scene — wife swapping, which particular world is well peopled with menopausal candidates. Illicit sexual liaisons achieve a magnetic appeal stronger than ever before — as does a wish for experimentation 'before it is too late'.

This factor is emphasised by Paul Rimmer who was the founder of the first English company to deal in sex aids. He was not reluctant to comment upon his own ageing process and paid really considerable tribute to his wife for the part she has played in keeping his sexual vigour at an appropriate level. He is now 56 and his comments are based on letters from customers together with his own personal experience.

There is no such thing as the male menopause physically. What it is, is a figure of speech covering the period of a man's life between the time he's growing old and the time he accepts that he is growing old.

No man has ever talked to me about the male menopause except as a joke — a jesting excuse for his behaviour or how he felt about things but never in earnest. It is all to do with accepting the fact that you are getting old — and of course, sex is the big thing. Men can accept that their hair is going grey and they haven't so many of their own teeth; that they can't run after a bus so quickly — but they find it difficult to accept that their sexual powers are going. Their egos are too much wrapped up in it. Their powers are waning in every way but this is the one way they can't accept. Eventually they have to and then I suppose they have come to the end of the so-called menopause.

The beginning is when they start to worry and it leads men to do some very odd things. For example, a lot of men experiment with homosexuality in their middle years. They are mainly respectable, straight married men. I don't think it is a case of latent homosexuality but a matter of trying anything that will give the man some sort of kick out of sex to bring back his virility.

Of course there is the chasing young girls thing too. I suppose all older men will look at young girls — and some older women look at young men — but wistfully. Very few men are fortunate enough to have had as full and varied a sex life as they would have liked. We would all like to have been Errol Flynns — and up to the time you're 40 there's still hope that if you push yourself out a bit maybe you can still do it all. But by the time there are grandchildren about it hits you — and that's when a lot of men start desperately trying to find a young mistress somewhere, anywhere. It's the women who get angry with their husbands making fools of themselves chasing young girls — but if he catches one he isn't such a fool . . . or is he?

It's just as big an ego boost for a woman at 45-50 to know that she's still wanted sexually by someone other than her husband. But if a woman is seen out with a younger man the response is that it isn't socially acceptable. She will be called a cradle snatcher and get herself laughed at, whereas with a man and a girl, people may sneer and say it's only his money, but there's a lot of envy and none of the stigma.

Of course, a lot of this is made much worse for the man and his so-called male menopause because it happens around the time of his wife's real one. Just at a time when he is beginning to feel all his own doubts and fears, his wife suddenly goes and behaves completely irrationally for a period of two to five years so he gets all these extra pressures when he is very vulnerable. He also gets the symptoms passed on to him by his wife — just like husbands with phantom pregnancies. Her nerves seem to be completely shattered at times and the same thing happens to his. The woman can become very insecure at that time, needing reassurance all the time, and what makes it worse is that the sexes don't understand one another very well.

Women don't understand how fragile men's egos are. Physically, in brute force, men may be much stronger than women but in every other way they are weaker. They are more romantic and less practical. Their egos can only too easily be shattered — and that comes home to roost quite unfairly when it comes to sex itself. The success of a sexual union seems to be still the responsibility of the man, particularly now that women are demanding that they should have as many orgasms as all those people who write to the sex magazines. The poor man is left carrying the burden which gets more and more difficult as he gets on and then comes this stage in middle life when his wife goes erratic and makes demands on him that he can't possibly fulfil.

Although men don't usually discuss their problems, especially sex, amongst themselves, they know in their own minds that they are all going through a period when they can't accept that they are cracking up — which they are, around 50. They are really going downhill. It's a period of bigger change for the worse than any other, obviously you start to go downhill very early on. But at first it is a gradual process, but in middle life it just seems to accelerate. I know it from my own experience. I'm not growing old gracefully. I do admit it — and I don't like it. Although I should know better. I've got all the hang-ups that most men have — and the main one is about losing my virility. But a lot of men give up very early on. I've known men of 40 who say, "Oh I'm finished. I'm not going to bother about sex any more." Certainly a lot of men my age have entirely lost interest in sex.

Frank Harris said that when he was a little boy his father gave him a pop gun to play with and when he was a little bit more sensible he gave him an air-gun. When he was a grown man, he taught him how to shoot and gave him a proper, lethal weapon. But, he goes on, the Good Lord gave him a lethal weapon to start with and the more he found out about how to use it, the more the Good Lord took it away and he ended up being an absolute expert with a little pop gun that was no use to anyone.

When a man is 45-50 and he suddenly realises that his potency is only half what it was 10 years earlier he immediately begins to worry and the worst thing he can do is worry — but how do you tell anyone not to worry? Most men have a failure some time in their lives. They go to bed and think everything is going to be OK but at the last minute it all collapses. Now, if you are a young man you think, "What the hell is the matter with me? Did I have too much to drink?" but you don't worry about it and by the next time you've forgotten it and everything is OK again. But when you're 45 you think, "This is the beginning of the end," and the next time you try it is still at the back of your mind and you are sub-consciously worrying. You can't will an erection and the more you think about it the less likely you are to get one. So it doesn't happen the second time and the third time it's worse. By then you are halfway gone so you go to the doctor and all kinds of things might happen. I've known of GP's who say, "You're 40 — what do you expect?" The GP can be as embarrassed as the patient — and often knows just as little. Or he might say, "Don't worry me with things like that. You're all right," and try to get rid of it as quickly as he can that way. Then he might say, "Just forget about it. Don't worry," but a man doesn't forget. He does worry. Too many men are worried and there just isn't enough money in medicine for it to be looked at properly — and the average GP doesn't consider it a matter of importance. But we see it from an entirely different viewpoint. Most of our customers are middle-aged people who have had a stable sexual relationship — married or otherwise — and they were trying to solve their problem together. And usually their difficulties are a combination of the female menopause and the so-called male menopause. That is why we have middle-aged men behind our counters and not young dolly birds. No man is going to discuss his sex problems with a girl young enough to be his daughter. Dolly girls only attract the tourists whereas a middle-aged man does inspire a certain amount of confidence if only because the customer knows that he may be going through the same problems himself.

A lot of men put it down to needing a change — to being in a rut. They think they need an injection of something new into their sex lives — and many of them do. They have got into a boring rut and then the male menopause as it were comes along and the thing gets worse and worse and they are flailing around looking for some sex aid that will help them. But once they're in that low and worried state there's not a lot a sex aid can do to help. The man needs to go with his partner to talk things over at a deeper personal, psychological level with some sensible sensitive person — if he's lucky enough to know one. I found that at least half my time in the shop was spent behind the desk talking to people about their problems — not selling things. Although I quite enjoyed it for part of the time, in the end it got too much. At times it made me feel so inadequate, not being able to help people. I could give them reassurance and that does some good, but in the last resort I'm not an expert or a therapist in that field.

Married men have their particular problems in coping if the condition strikes them so that they feel forced to find extra-marital outlets. Often, their situation is exacerbated by their anxieties about all the deceptions required to prevent exposure to the world at large or their wives and families. Bachelors are not, however, immune, and two personal testimonies follow from unmarried men.

The first is from a man who suffered — in his own perception — very badly from the male menopause. Happily, he is one of those who have overcome it and we are delighted to be able to include not only his view of what happened to him while he was still a victim but also a letter he was good enough to write to us outlining his suggested approaches for any man who wanted to cure or prevent it. The letter is to be found on p.157.

I'm 46 now and out of it, but for the two years, when I was 43 and 44, the menopause was terrible. My behaviour was very odd and I suspected that I was going quite dotty. I started to shout at people in the street about the way they dropped litter. I carried on a tremendous campaign in a most unreasonable fashion about a road sign that had no light inside it. A friend of mine had had an accident at the junction and I kept on complaining to the police. I spent an inordinate amount of time and attention on it, even pestering the council. I also used to shout at women who allowed their dogs to foul the pavements. I was tetchy and over-responsive to little things.

I was trying to put myself straight by shouting at the world and suddenly I could see myself stumping along with a stick — the middle-aged type who declares war! Then a woman friend of mine who was about 60 at the time started to get on my nerves and I treated her very badly — my behaviour was quite unreasonable. She said, "The trouble with you is you're going through the male menopause." Now at the time I thought it was a typically bitchy, childish thing to say but it stuck in my mind, and after a time I was able to stand back and note what was happening to me. The minute I did that I found that a close friend of mine of similar age and temperament was also behaving in a terrible manner and he hadn't realised it either. Then I heard that another friend — whom I hadn't known all that well when we were young — was in a most unhappy state in America. He had bought an estate outside Chicago which was supposed to bring him idyllic happiness but it hadn't turned out that way, so I wrote to him.

It was the equivalent of recreating the past, my early 20's, and I was also supposed to be helping somebody — which in my mind is always a straightforward give-away that you're really attempting to help yourself. We wrote to each other quite a lot over these two years and I became a sort of village elder, all by post. They were long letters. Mine were much the longer and in the end I must have told him the whole story of my life. I don't think he got all that much help out of it because he's a much more isolated person than I am, very introverted and pessimistic. I'm more on the ball, so, by putting my own feelings into words, I began to understand myself much better.

Likewise with my other friend, Frank, who was also behaving very oddly, through analysing him I understood myself better. He had an absolute obsession about immigrants. He is a most tolerant person and not given to prejudice generally, but when it came to this area — and only at this time — he became unbelievably biased and vicious. He would call them niggers, coons and gollies. Everything is due to the gollies he would say. He's got over all that now and is also much better. However, at the time it made it easier for me to identify, to recognise myself and to admit, "I've got this obsession about that traffic light or what have you."

Professional and financial troubles seemed to be mounting as well. Looking back I can see that there were problems but not as many nor of the stature I thought. Everything seemed to come all at once — personal, professional and financial. Suddenly I was no longer 25 and it mattered, I could feel time passing and I found adjustment to middle age very daunting. I suppose I could have coped with all these things if I had been in a normal state — but you never know which comes first, what causes which. For a time it centred on the Inland Revenue. I seemed to be getting, willy-nilly, letters from them in those awful buff envelopes. I used to leave them around unopened for days on end. I moved them from place to place and then I would actually hide them. In the end, with each one, I would take a dose of tranquillisers and ring up friends and say, "Will you come and stay with me while I open it?" My heart used to beat faster and I would feel dreadful — trembling all over. And then it got so that I dreaded the post in the mornings — any letters, no matter what they said. Now it's completely different. I look forward to the post again and I don't even mind the buff envelopes. I'm able to feel, "Take me to court if you want to; put me in a debtors' prison if you want to." But I couldn't do any of that three years ago. I couldn't have talked as I am doing now. I would have drawn all the curtains and hidden away. I've done that many times. I couldn't bear to talk to strangers about the way I was feeling — not face to face anyway. I would ring the Samaritans in the middle of the night and tell them that my life had no meaning and no purpose and, "Why were all these people alive anyway? It just doesn't make sense." I couldn't understand any of it. The Samaritans advised me to find someone to love but I kept saying, "You can't love anybody else unless you love yourself." And I didn't love myself . . . I had somehow to find myself first.

I didn't see any point in living but I didn't decide to kill myself because that would have upset my parents and friends — and people who had faith in me. It would have destroyed too many things for no good reason. It seems crazy to me now that I could even have thought about it, but at the time I had absolutely nothing to live for. It was ludicrous and only by examining everything in the minutest detail did I manage to get things into perspective. For example, I found that I had let the flat go to rack and ruin. I had done nothing to it for months. I realised then that I had made my bed but not bothered to make it — and it was the one I was lying on, the one I was stuck with because it wasn't just my bed, it was my life.

Slowly I began to realise I had to lower my sights and to compromise. When I was young I was going to be Shakespeare: I was going to be the greatest writer on earth. People were literally going to fall back in amazement and exclaim, "You must be the man who wrote so-and-so." Whenever I signed a hotel register people would recognise my name. I would live permanently in the South of France and wear white shoes. They were really banal dreams! I now no longer want those dreams anyway, but, more importantly, I have realised that part of the getting older process is to stop having dreams and to get rid of ambitions. It's much easier to live without them. The early sacrifices I made to be a writer were awful. Going through this menopausal crisis has taught me that I wouldn't do it now. I've realised now that the trick is to stop trying so hard to do everything not only well but superlatively well, and life is much easier. It's all much less anxious now that I don't feel I have to prove myself any more. I'm not always testing myself against the world as I did before. I've stopped worrying about confidence. I don't know whether I've found it or not but it doesn't seem to matter now. Before I was very shy and never able to say what I felt. I was caught by the inhibitions that had been forced into me by my genteel middle class background. Now I no longer care what people think — or perhaps to be more realistic, I don't think I care what people think. This was an important breakthrough for me since it meant that I could drop people who bored me or burdened me. Now I'm able to say, "Go to a doctor. Go to a clinic. I'm not a therapist or a counsellor." It's not at all sympathetic or kind in the clichéd meanings of those words I know, but I decided that I had my own problems and that I wasn't going to be burdened. All I want to hear now is good news and happy endings. Friends have pursued me — even the ones I tried really hard to drop. "It's impossible to get you on the phone," they would say. One old girl friend I'd known for years who was terribly boring, eventually wrote a card in desperation. It ended, "Don't you want to be friends any more?" — I just didn't answer it. To tell the truth, I didn't want to be friends and that was just too bad I thought. I've been dropped in my time so I know the score — but it's ridiculous carrying burdens and calling them relationships.

During the middle of it all I had a different kind of dream — but no less stupid and unrealistic than the ones of my youth. I was going to run away and live by the sea with a little garden. I was going to retire from life and hide from it all in an isolated farmhouse. Now that's a common dream and it doesn't work either. I discovered that you can't just become a mild middle class gent. Another dream was to give up my career in writing and open a school. There was a possibility that my landlord might buy me out and I would use the money to start up this project. I'm glad now that I didn't . And, in any case, it was ridiculous because I'd be useless as an administrator — and, more ridiculous still, I was absolutely incapable of communicating with anybody at all — in a positive way that is. There was this painter friend of mine from years back. He's been like a brother in fact. Every year he comes to stay with me at least twice for a longish period. He visited me when I was suffering from this menopause and I behaved with terrible pettiness towards him. I offered him unbelievable malice. He was terribly hurt and puzzled at first because I really was evil. I would come downstairs and, if he'd left a coffee cup out of place, I would scream and slam out of the place so that the door would make the flat shake and I would make enough noise to awaken the neighbourhood. I knew I was doing it but I couldn't do anything to stop it. When he confronted me about it I used to burst into tears. There seemed to be no person of any kind who could help me at all. The Samaritans were in their way the most helpful since I didn't really see them as people. It was easier to talk to them than it was to close friends, acquaintances or anybody that I thought was remotely real.

Work was another factor that helped me to get through it. I suddenly got an important big commission and this meant I didn't have the time to devote to my grim state. I was listless and I didn't particularly want to work but the commission was there and I had accepted it so I got on with it night and day while meantime the menopause went on and on and I thought, "It will pass. Nature will cure you in the end. It can't get any worse than this."

A strange thing is that when you are pathetic, the more helpless you are, the more attractive you are to other people — many of them anyway. It would seem that helplessness is the most attractive quality a person can have. Throughout the whole period there was never a shortage of sexual partners. Women were just as interested in me as they'd always been and one would think that might have fed my vanity but it was no comfort whatsoever. It gave me no gratification of any kind.

I didn't lose or put on weight. My teeth didn't fall out and my hair didn't go. It's thinning a bit but that's of no consequence. Physically I was still the healthy specimen I'd always been. There was no decline of any kind that I noticed in physical things — although I have read that men have hormonal changes too. Their skin may become coarser and less resilient in the way that a woman's does at the same time, with the hair getting grey and that sort of thing, but none of that happened to me. But it was still no help to know that.

What really helped me in the end was helping other people and I made some lovely new friends during the period of the abyss and that was much more reassuring than any sexual or intellectual attractiveness I might still have had. I kept the depressed side of myself from my new friends as much as I could — letting that come out only when I was with, say, Frank. But as for actually talking much about me and what was happening, that I could only do with the people who seemed to need help in the same areas themselves. During the whole of that time I had no sexual interest of any kind. It all went. As it happens I'm bi-sexual but I became completely apathetic about the whole thing — men and women. It wouldn't even have made any difference if you'd brought Marilyn Monroe herself into my bed. But I wasn't worried about it. I've never had any period of sexual impotence at all thank God. I've had times when I didn't feel like sex, perhaps for a month at a time, but that's just a normal part of life. It happens often when I have a lot of work to do. But going to bed with someone doesn't help when you're in the sort of predicament that I was. It wouldn't have helped at all — the suffering of the condition is all that you can be concerned about. Flailing about looking for sexual partners is certainly not the answer.

Whether things might have been different if I'd married I don't know. All my life I've found it very easy to attract people who want me as a sexual partner and I haven't thought of marriage as a realistic possibility since I was in my twenties. There was a girl then who was in the throes of divorce and we planned to marry but it didn't come about. I think I was more upset than she was but there were too many problems — too many people involved. In the end she got her divorce and married someone else and is even now still happy I believe. I have never wanted to marry anybody since then. It gets more difficult as you get older. You do get set in your ways and although there is a constant circuit of younger women after older men I find that they bore me. I'm more concerned with the qualities of kindness and assurance that I find in slightly older women. They are much more important than physical attributes.

Having come through it all now, I can sympathise with my mother much more than I could when she was having her menopause. She did some pretty strange things and I didn't understand at all. I remember her getting herself up in the most terribly vivid, lurid outfits and I thought, "What on earth is she wearing that for?" She looked like a whore and behaved in exactly the same ways that I did when it was at its worst. With my father it was more disguised since he lived his life in a permanent anxiety state — but there's no doubt they suffered . . . as I did.

The next contribution is also from an unmarried man. He is a homosexual, but unlike Quentin Crisp, he does not see the future holding anything but despair and tragedy for him. He sees himself caught in an ever-closing cage and trap — without hope for escape or relief.

Three or four years ago I slipped a disc. "That's a sure sign of middle age," I thought and I went to this ancient medico at a hospital and he said, "Well; it's what you have to expect. You are, after all, coming up for the meen-o-pause." I just thought, "Christ."

I'm a homosexual so it's a much worse problem for me. You've got no offspring, no progeny. You're in danger of imminent termination — the end of the line — full stop. The normal family man doesn't suffer in the same way. At least he has made his mark and his life won't be a write-off. He has some children to show for it all. Being homosexual you haven't got that. It's all inadequacy and hopelessness. But by far the worse problem is impotence in intercourse. It's really very bad indeed. I can never get an orgasm during sexual intercourse these days, only through masturbation. Of course I'm not sure how much of this is to do with my menopause and how much it would have happened anyway. But I got so worried about it that I mentioned it to a shrink. I go to one occasionally when I'm feeling particularly bad. About my impotence he said it might have to do with the slipped disc — that it had affected my nervous system. I don't know about that but I still worry. I hate it. What happens is that I have an erection, it hovers around for a bit — and then at the vital moment it disappears. Now, if this had happened thirty to thirty-five years ago I wouldn't have minded all that much. I would have been sure that I had plenty of time and plenty of partners left. But now I'm 52 I don't have a lot of time left for sex. I know that time is running out — and I love sex.

On top of all that, I haven't done half the things I've wanted to do creatively as a composer, and I just can't reconcile myself to it. With the menopause coming on you think, "Life's more than halfway through," and I'm frightened that I won't be able to pack in what I have in mind. That's what I can't come to terms with. Being a homosexual is bad enough. It took a lot of courage some years ago when I decided that I would come out in the open and admit, "Yes, I am a homosexual." That in itself is a terrible thing to bear. It leaves you with a tremendous feeling of inadequacy. It's all very well talking about our permissive society but there's still so much stigma attached to being a homosexual that life's often pretty hellish. And the age thing is even more important too. In the queer world it's an unmitigated crime to be more than 25. I just daren't let it be known how old I am. One of my lovers the other day was scornful of a man he'd met who wanted to sleep with him. He said to me, "He was at least 50 years old. He was really old!" My blood ran cold — he has no idea I am 52. It's an incredibly cold, cruel harsh world that homosexuals live in. That's why I can't possibly allow my name to be exposed. I'd be attacked for having the male menopause and for my impotence — and in the most ruthless cruel way.

On the other hand, during the last five years I have had quite extra-ordinary love affairs, three of them at a very deep level. You know what they say, "When you think you are past love, 'tis then you find your last love"? But although the love itself has been splendid I haven't had an orgasm in partnership with anybody else for a long time. Two of the men were heterosexuals. I tend to go for them rather than homosexuals — they are not so obsessed with youth as homosexuals are. Queers absolutely have to have young people. For myself, given a free range, I really go for Oriental men; men with smooth hairless bodies. And I get very cheesed off when I'm not getting what I want regulalry and frequently, so decline in sexual attraction and performance does affect me very badly indeed. It's no exaggeration to say there is a geriatric syndrome in the homosexual world. You're very quickly on the scrap heap and since all my *affaires* are with young men — I'm only attracted to young men — things look very bad for me. The only man of my own age I've ever slept with is a man I've known for twenty years. He's Japanese and looks about 20 until you really look closely at his face and see the lines. But even he has the smooth skin, the body of a young man and the very thick hair.

Needless to say, he dyes it. I don't dye mine but I do use all sorts of lotions and things to make it grow. They don't work of course! Nothing really works and here am I terrified of finding myself in the position of nobody wanting to put their arms around me any more. That's the really frightening thing. And the fear comes at a time when you've no reserves to cope with it, because there are all the physical things as well. One simply isn't as fit physically any more. You seem to plod rather than run around. You never have a light spring in the toes any more. I find that I'm gasping for breath at the top of the stairs. When I was young and used to get pissed I was as right as rain the next day. Now I feel dreadful. The body no longer has the same power to make up for such things. Your eyesight goes and there's a terrible deterioration in the quality of your skin. You get aches in your limbs. If you bend down to do something, you can't spring up like you used to. And then weight! From when I was about 17 to a few years ago I was ten stone seven pounds, and then I started drinking. I seemed to spend a whole year drinking and I put on two stone and I've never been able to lose it. The only time I lost any at all was when one of my lovers left me and I went terribly thin and got very suicidal. I've bought a bicycle to try to lose weight and I go out on it at least once a day.

Then there's the brain. Your memory goes. I can't remember words any more — and names are terrible. The other day I was writing to someone I know quite well and I couldn't remember his surname. "Roger, Roger," I kept saying but the surname wouldn't come. And the trouble is that for a homosexual there is no compensation. I've never met a happy homosexual. There's no such thing.

The most galling factor is that I haven't made it and so I think, "What went wrong; and is the pattern for the next, the last twenty five years?" I know the work I do is good — but on too many occasions now no inspiration comes. When you're young, you don't mind. It's all in front of you. It's all ahead, all anticipation. But now that 'AHEAD' is behind me. When the future is in front of you anything can happen — but my future is now behind me and it hasn't happened. That is an appalling reality to have to contend with. I wake up in the middle of the night and the cold truth dawns. I get depressed and I can't work and then my income plummets as well. I get into a state of despair and then spend so much time looking for sex and it is time and energy that should be poured into my work — not diverted into searching for sex. And as for the old myth that an artist should suffer if he is any good, it's simply not true. A good artist is a happy one, and I'm not that. At my age I should be established. You can tolerate not being established when you're young, but not at 52. So the older I get the more important sex becomes. I'm driven in a way no man should be — frightened of ageing and terrified of dying. That's why I have to have young friends. My quid pro quo with them is that I give them something from my knowledge and experience and they keep me in touch with their *élan vital,* and I desperately need that. You see, a heterosexual man who is married has living proof of his virility, living proof of his own immortality in his children.

I desperately wanted children. At one time I might have had children but now I accept that it isn't going to happen — or at least I try to. One's whole life is a preparation for death and if you haven't learned to cope with it by the time you're my age, it's pretty grim. I've just got to find out how to face it.

Once, when I was pretty neurotic about it, I went to this doctor — he's some kind of psychiatrist associated with the IBA — and told him what was troubling me and he gave me some pills. When I got home I read on the bottle that they were not to be taken if you were eating certain foods. The warning suggested that the results could be fatal. I thought, "Christ, I'd better not take these pills without seeing this doctor again." So I made another appointment and asked him about them. He was furious. He showed me the door and told me to get out and stop wasting his time. I was totally shattered. At the very time when I needed some understanding from a professional who was supposed to be in that special field, he turned me away.

Of course, the ideal situation — one that I've thought, written and composed about a lot — would be for older queers always to live with younger men. And then when they died the young man would be older and would in turn choose a young man of his own. It's only a pipe dream of course — and I know I have nothing as happy as that to look forward to.

Some men get caught by their need to experiment sexually and become voyeurs and exhibitionists. Some find themselves trying homosexual liaisons just for the kicks they think they might get — but others discover a previously buried genuine desire for a homosexual relationship. An apparently normal heterosexual man may undergo a transformation of his needs and suddenly find himself gripped by powerful homosexual tendencies. The hero of Thomas Mann's novel *Death in Venice* finds himself passionately enamoured of a young man and demonstrates the terrible, tragic consequences that such a dramatic switch can bring about.

From what we have been told, we believe that when a menopausal man begins to experience the desperation of desiring sex with a man 'just this once' he can only too easily become racked by a 'Now or Never' need which may lead him into many unthinking excesses — which in turn carry him into a world overshadowed by all kinds of social threats. Indulgences of this kind often bring much more disastrous consequences than a fling with a young girl. After all, he has been there before and does know something about the rules, the roles and the ropes, and while he may be in danger of losing his sense of direction, he is at least not doing so in an alien country.

There is the additional problem that he may discover that he is more homosexual than heterosexual and intercourse with his wife may become repugnant to him. Should his wife learn the reason for this disaffection it could be a shattering blow for her — far more difficult to overcome than being superceded by a young woman. She too could get easily lost in a sexual and emotional world that is completely new to her. She may feel desolate and sexually and socially degraded — quite incapable of mentioning the matter to her GP or her confidantes. Thus she could become isolated in her emotions and sexually devalued at a time when she also may need special understanding and more, not less, supportive affection and desire. Certainly she will not be put in a position where it will be easy for her to help her husband — even if he should ask for her help.

Not many men actually turn to homosexual relationships. The best known symptom, and probably the most frequent, is the search for a revitalising relationship with a young woman. The only thing that seems capable of bringing some men back to life is the feel of a full young breast under their ageing palms:

"She stood, a sight to make an old man young."

And it is well-known throughout history — especially in the Old Testament, that ever-faithful stand-by for lustful chauvinists — that old men who could afford to pay the price, have warmed their beds and attempted to warm their hearts, minds and bodies through the possession of young girls. But with them, as with the menopausal man today, no young woman's body can compensate for that sexual frigidity or secondary impotence that stems from deprivation and inadequacy. Only the man can do that for himself. James Hemming points out (on p.154) that a wise woman might be able to re-orientate a man undergoing a menopausal crisis. We are not quite so optimistic as that, believing that every man does what *he* wants to do and that none of us can hope to find salvation in the person or advice of another — and the menopausal man is the same: he must find his own step-ladder from the abyss he has himself dug.

Instead of gaining the enjoyment he may well be entitled to from his actual achievements (home, family, leisure and work interests — which most potential victims have to some degree) many a man would sacrifice most of what he has for a week or two (perhaps as little as a weekend) in the South of France with a rapaciously sexy young thing. This may well be the case if sexual relationships with his wife have been tame or non-existent. Such a circumstance is a breeding ground for an obsession with young girls' bodies before the dreaded impotence sets in. (Naturally the question must be asked: Why were sexual relationships not as they might have been — and in the answer may lie many of the causes for the man's menopausal state.)

Some men lack the necessary confidence and courage to exercise their charms on the open socio-sexual market where they fear they may not score. They are likely to turn to prostitutes, call-girls and masseuses, knowing that they will not be rejected; confident there is no 'competition'; and secure in their belief that they will be offered full professional boosting for their flagging egos. Not all men can overcome their feelings of guilt about such relationships and can bring themselves to achieve no more than a visit to a night club for a close dancing session with a hostess — or, failing that, an evening at a strip club where finally they may resort to masturbation to convince themselves that they are still OK. As a last resort, some men will turn to the pages of the girlie magazines for the apparently seductive consolations of the paper girls.

Even this area is not without its attendant hazards. Although we have in many ways approval for many of the women who earn their living by selling their bodies (as opposed to many of us who sell our souls and pay the price for the social dry cleaning that is required to keep us in our states of whited sepulchres) there are some who cheat and not all menopausal men are equipped to recognise them, or to do anything about it once they discover the fraud. Such an experience can be a torment for some men. Others get so much pleasure and such a boost from their experiences that they get well and truly hooked on the hookers, and we have many cases of men who have spent thousands of pounds chasing their lost youth in the arms of call-girls. Provided they can afford it, we find little harm here since their relationships with their wives must have reached such a low ebb that they are past reclaim. But trouble really sets in when the man cannot afford what he desperately feels he needs from these girls and this can cause the meno-pausal bank assistant or solicitor to turn to theft. The consequences of such an action are obvious — the man losing a job, a way of life, which he may have spent his best years creating. Just like youth and virility, he will only see the value in this way of life, or profession, once it has gone.

Even on the open socio-sexual market there are snags and pitfalls. The man may succeed in attracting a young girl . . . and then spend the rest of the relationship waiting in terror for her to tire of him although he may have jeopardised a marriage of many years' standing just to caress her firm young body. His temporary rejuvenation may be at the cost of this rack of fear as well as his guilt feelings regarding his wife. There may also be the totally ambivalent feelings he may experience because his new-found mistress is younger than his daughters. When the first *hot flush* of his sexual passion has been cooled in the winds of reality (be they gentle breezes or destructive gales) he may discover he has lost the final vestige of self-respect through behaving 'badly' according to his own standards as well as those whose opinion he cares about. But he may still be too intoxicated to give up what varies from a mere dalliance to an habitual indulgence or a total infatuation.

His wife may not be able to get a lover of her own so easily and, even if she could, may have no desire to do so, and this may make the man's unfairness to her clearer for him to see. One consequence of this is that his guilt grows and manifests itself in many ways from explosively bitter tempers to bribes of expensive holidays and prodigal gifts.

Ironically, the better his wife and her behaviour during this period (demonstrating her understanding, empathy and compassion perhaps) the worse is the man likely to feel about what he is doing; his wife; and his marriage. He would much prefer her to give him appropriate justification (in his eyes) by behaving towards him in a way that he could represent as lacking in understanding — the "My wife doesn't understand me" syndrome.

Once **having** started on the slippery slope of infidelity, the man may find it difficult or impossible to stop. His thin-skinned bubble of sexual reputation will be in need of constant care and attention. One mistress can so quickly lead to another and the man gets on the self-defeating band-waggon of quantity when his only escape route lies in the pursuit of quality. He is deluded and so measures fulfilment in pounds of flesh when he should be seeking ounces of integrity. Quantity may, for a strictly limited period, quieten his aching symptoms, whereas quality would help him approach the cause — and so enable him to get at least into striking distance of dignity. Then, and only then, might he retain or regain some good feelings about himself and his behaviour patterns.

An affaire with a young girl brings another dangerous complexity into the arena. If the man begins to over-value the 'meat-market' aspect of young girls' bodies, he may well go off sex with his wife. It is not easy for a middle-aged woman to compete with the body of a lithe young girl. (The fact that her husband should not require this kind of assessment of virtue or genius-of-self is no comfort or help since that is the standard he will hold dear — and it is not easy for a wife to convince him he is wrong when so much money is spent on advertising the fact that he is right.) It is never easy for a wife to compete on such grounds, even at the best of times — and a menopausal male of the carnally minded, chauvinistic kind is at the worst of times. He will set up the competitive situation exclusively on the grounds of youth, glamorously made-up 'good' looks, and in all probability, big breasts — all symbols and symptoms of the man's anxieties about his insecure external image.

Although he may continue intercourse (all possibilities of *making love* are more than likely to have flown) with his wife, it will be out of a sense of duty or motivated by guilt, and this will do nothing but compound his problems since it is not impossible that he will now become impotent with his wife. Whether this is from physical distaste, shame and guilt, sexual over-indulgence elsewhere or a combination of all of these will not affect it exacerbating his situation and perhaps becoming the final straw that breaks his relationship with his wife or harms one or both of them beyond easy recovery.

No matter how distasteful a knowledge of the man's sexual pro-clivities may be to his wife at this time, it is possible that she will be able to understand them, if not actually forgive. When the symptoms pile up in the form of apparently unprompted and uncalled-for depressions or bouts of over-active tension and mental stress, the wife may have no conception of what is happening to her menopausal husband. The attacks can build up to powerful indeed monumental proportions and we believe there is a good case for examining the incidence of suicide and attempted suicide at this time in men's lives.

Let us turn to the victims themselves to find out what it feels like experientially when the menopausal condition strikes in such a way. First Colin Wilson, perhaps still best known for *The Outsider*, describes how he fought attacks that came in waves.

When I was young, T S Eliot told me the way to survive personally and as a writer was to start by becoming known to a small circle of people and gradually increase the size so that it never got out of hand — not to make an impact in a big way with a mass audience to begin with. I did it the other way round and learned to my cost that he was right.

Daphne du Maurier also said that if you make a big hit with a book — or anything indeed — when you are young, the chances are that you will go through a decade when you are virtually ignored.

My name was mud from 1956 to 1971 which is a hell of a long time — and during the whole of that period I had no help with my writing at all. So from being at the top I began a slow descent — a running down — and when I was asked to do an Arts programme with Westward Television I actually went to pieces in front of the camera. I found that I'd been going round in my head for so long that I couldn't face the reality of people any more.

A lot of people get breakdowns in their 40's. Some even die. What happens is that you've packed so much into life until that time — then suddenly you are no longer young. Suddenly you realise that you are galloping on to 50 and 60. This knowledge reduces your motivation just as it does for a woman at her menopause. If you get through it, I think you have a good chance of going on and thriving. But when it strikes — in the 40's as it does — it strikes with a force that can provoke panic or paralysis.

At the time when I was still collecting material for *'Mysteries'*, I had a nasty but curiously fascinating experience: a series of attacks of 'panic anxiety' that brought me close to a nervous breakdown. What surprised me most was that I was not depressed or worried at the time. I was working hard — very hard — but I seemed to be taking it all in my stride. For the past eighteen months, I had been involved on the editorial board of a kind of encyclopedia of crime; but every meeting ended in disagreement, and it began to look as if the whole project would have to be abandoned. Then, at short notice, the publisher decided to go ahead. Suddenly, everything had to be completed in a few months; and I, as coordinator, was asked to produce around a hundred articles — 3,000 words each — at a rate of about seven a week. I began to work at the typewriter for eight or nine hours a day, and tried to unwind in the evenings.

One day, a couple of journalists came to interview me. They booked into a nearby hotel, and came to supper. They were young and enthusiastic, with a tendency to interrupt one another. By the time they left, at about two in the morning, my eyes were glazed, and I was feeling slightly deafened. This, I later realised, was the trouble. When you become bored, you 'let yourself go'; you sink into a kind of moral torpor, and cease to make any effort. The next day, they came back for another session with the tape recorder. When they left, I felt too dull to do any writing; instead, I took the opportunity to perform a number of routine household tasks. And that night, at about 4 a.m., I woke up feeling unrested, and began to think about all the other articles I still had to write, and the books I ought to be writing instead. Anxiety hormones trickled into my bloodstream, and my heart began to beat too fast. I felt a desire to get up now and go to my typewriter although I realised it would be more sensible to get some sleep. Lying there, with nothing else to think about, made it worse. It was rather like feeling physically sick; and when it was clear that I was not going to improve things by ignoring it, I tried making a frontal assault, and suppressing it by sheer concentration. That proved to be a mistake. My face became hot, and I felt a dangerous tightness across the chest, while my heartbeat accelerated to a point that terrified me. I got up, went to the kitchen, and poured myself a glass of orange juice. Then I sat down, and tried to calm myself, as I might soothe a frightened horse. Gradually, I got it under control, and went back to bed. But as soon as I was in the dark, it started again: rising panic, accelerating heartbeat, the feeling of being trapped. This time I got up and went into the sitting room. I was inclined to wonder if I was having a heart attack. The panic kept rising like vomit; the calm, sane part of me kept saying it was absurd, some minor physical problem that would solve itself within twenty four hours. It came in waves, every few minutes, and in between each wave, there was a brief feeling of calm and relief.

The worst thing was the fear that this could escalate until all my energy was gone, like milk boiling over in a saucepan. The anxiety produced panic; the panic produced further anxiety — a fear *of* fear. It seemed that any move I made to counter the fear could in turn be negated by the fear. In theory, the fear could overrule every attempt I made to overrule it. On the other hand, although this was a kind of nausea, I was aware that it would be no solution to give way to it, as you can safely give way to physical nausea and allow yourself to vomit. This fear was destructive, like a forest fire, and had to be contained.

I *had* experienced something of the sort, long before; but without this sense of physical danger. One day at school, a group of us had been discussing where space ended, and I was suddenly shocked to realise that this seemed to be an *unanswerable* question. It struck me that I had always felt secure because I had taken it for granted that this universe is logical and rational, and that someone, somewhere, knew all the answers. Now I recognised that grown-ups are in this respect no better than children, and the thought produced a kind of dizziness, like falling. For years afterwards, the feeling would recur, especially in crowds, the realisation that human beings are living in a fool's paradise, comfortably enmeshed in their little values and incapable of seeing beyond them. The same thought occurred to me one day when I saw a sheep feeding its lambs, looking a picture of motherly solicitude, unaware that she and her lambs were destined for someone's oven.

Now, as I sat in the armchair and tried to repress the panic, I knew it was important not to start thinking about these basic questions: of our total ignorance, of our lack of the smallest shred of certainty about who we are and why we are here. That way, I realised, lay insanity, a fall into a kind of mental 'black hole'.

I suppose what seemed most ironical was that I had always felt I understood the causes of mental illness. A couple of years before, I had written a book called *New Pathways in Psychology,* in which I had argued that all mental illness is due to the collapse of the will. When you are making an effort, your will recharges your vital powers as a car recharges its battery when you drive it. If you cease to will, the battery goes flat, and life appears to be futile and absurd. To emerge from this state, all that is necessary is to maintain *any* kind of purposeful activity — even without much conviction — and the batteries will slowly become recharged. That is what I had said. And now, struggling with this panic, all the certainty had vanished. Instead, I found myself thinking of my novel *The Mind Parasites,* in which I had suggested that there are creatures that live in the depths of our subconscious minds, draining our vitality like leeches. That seemed altogether closer to what I was now experiencing.

Finally, I felt sufficiently calm — and cold — to go back to bed. I lay there, staring at the grey square of the window, glad that some automatic resistance had awakened in me, and hoping that the daylight would make the whole thing seem as unimportant as a bad dream. In fact, I woke up feeling low and exhausted, and at the back of my mind there was a feeling as if I had received some appalling bad news. I worked through the day, and the effort made me feel better. But in the evening, I felt drained, and the fear began to return. I watched a television programme, and felt myself sinking into depression as into a swamp. I would make an effort, rouse myself to mental activity, and suddenly feel better. Then something in the programme would 'remind' me of the fear; there was a kind of inner jerk, like a car slipping out of gear, and the sinking feeling was back.

The articles still had to be written; in fact, a few days later, the editor rang me to ask if I could produce ten during the next week, instead of seven. An American backer was waving his chequebook and demanding speed. Since I had already decided against the temptation to back out of the project, I stepped up my production to an article and a half a day. I was treating myself like a man with snake-bite, forcing myself to keep walking. Gradually, I began to learn the tricks of this strange war against myself. One of the worst attacks came three months later, on a sleeper train from London. The panic became so overpowering that I was afraid I might suffer cardiac arrest. At one point, I seriously considered getting off the train at the next stop and walking, no matter where. Then, in one of the periodic ebbs of panic, I forced myself to repeat a process I had taught myself in previous attacks: to reach inside myself and try to untie the mental knots. While I was doing this, it struck me that if I could soothe myself from panic into 'normality', then surely there was no reason why I shouldn't soothe myself *beyond* normality, into a still deeper state of calm? I made this effort, and felt the inner turmoil gradually subside. Until the spasms ceased; then I pressed on, breathing deeply, inducing still deeper relaxation. My breathing became shallow, and almost ceased. Suddenly, it was as if a boat had been lifted off a sandbank by the tide; I felt a kind of inner jerk, and floated into a state of deep quiescence. When I thought about this, later the same day, it struck me that I had achieved a state that is one of the basic aims of yoga; Rilke's 'stillness like the heart of a rose.'

After the first two or three attacks, I began to understand their basic mechanism. To begin with, there was the old problem of self-consciousness. If you think about itching, you begin to itch. If you think about feeling sick, you feel sick. Consciousness directed back on itself produces the 'amplification effect'. If I woke up in the middle of the night. I often slipped into a state of self-consciousness that would trigger the panic mechanism. I had to perfect the trick of 'thinking about something else'. Once I had learned to do this, the attacks became easier to avert.

But when I tried to go to the heart of the problem, I had to acknowledge that my trouble was a certain basic 'childishness'. When a child is pushed beyond a certain limit of fatigue or tension, its will surrenders. Some instinctive sense of fair-play is outraged, and it declines to make any further effort. An adult may feel like surrendering to a problem, but common sense and stubbornness force the will to further effort. As an obsessive worker, I am accustomed to drive myself hard. Experience has taught me that when I get over-tired, the quickest way to recovery is often to drive myself on until I get 'second wind'. But to do this effectively, you need the full support of your subconscious mind. In this case, I was trying to push myself beyond my normal limits, and some childish element in my subconscious had gone on strike. It was sitting with folded arms and a sullen expression, declining to do its proper work of recharging my vital batteries. And so, when I passed beyond a certain point of fatigue, I would suddenly discover there was no more energy to call on. It was like descending a ladder and discovering that the last half dozen rungs are missing. At which point, I had to force my conscious mind to interfere: a thing it is reluctant to do, since the subconscious usually knows best. I had to tell myself sternly that I was being bloody stupid; that in my younger days, I worked far harder as a navvy or machine operator than I have ever worked as a writer, and that writing for a living has made me lazy and spoilt.

The panic, then, was caused by a lower level of my being, an incompetent and immature 'me'. While I identified with this 'me', I was in danger. But the panic could always be averted by waking myself up fully and calling upon a more purposive 'me'. The moment it appeared, it was like a schoolmistress walking into a room full of squabbling children, and clapping her hands. The panic would subside instantly, to be succeeded by a sheepish silence.

And now perhaps one of the most dramatic cases of all. We have already mentioned that John Bratby had painted a portrait involving Lucan and Stonehouse in his protrayal of the male menopause and the use of another of John's portraits on the cover suggests that he might have an unexpected interest in the subject. His description of what occurred is graphic and frightening — and something of a sober warning for those who condescendingly smile or just shrug off the idea that the male menopause is a force to be reckoned with.

The sort of traumas that are associated with the male menopause can drive you mad. You may not appear to be mad, not outwardly, but they can drive you right out of your mind.

Looking back to my parents' situation it now seems perfectly obvious that they split because of both their cases of menopausal troubles. They went their separate ways and soon after that, they were both dead. My father died at about 50 and my mother earlier. In the beginnings of the marriage it was all more than happy and then the menopausal situation came along for both. And there are photographs where the faces of the children show that they were badly affected by the situation.

My mother died of a ruptured spleen and my father died of pneumonia, but of course when the mind gives up the body gives up as well. It doesn't resist the onset of disease. And it seems to me that they'd just given up mentally.

Their pattern is very clear to me now. It all fits — although I didn't know it at the time. And my own case echoes it as I look back at what happened to them.

Just before the break — break-up or breakdown, it's all the same, and I prophesied it in my novel, prophesied it all — all the things had been built up in life. The material things had been gained. The house had been decorated inside and out. One had a very expensive car and everything was achieved, and then without realising it you look to the future and nothing is there.

I seem to see so many examples of it around. Around about the time it happened to me there was a man — my son visited his home — and he was very successful with two factories. All the material things were there, big house, Jensen, etcetera, very rich . . . the man had worked twenty years to achieve everything he had . . . yet there was no communication between the man and his wife any more and he was to be seen coming home rolling drunk. And, as I understand it, this is what often happens. All the material goals are achieved with all the energies of the late 20's and 30's and then you start to look around and there's nothing to go for any more. You don't realise what's happening to you at the particular point except that everything has gone stale and it shouldn't have because you've got everything you wanted. This is in the material area but in my case there was the artistic area and that was something else.

In my case I was painting for a one man exhibition and I found myself painting a 25 year old lady from the Royal College of Art and that broke the marriage, the family and the home up. The break was caused by a catalyst . . . somebody comes along at the right time and the break happens. I thought I'd fallen desperately in love with her. But when you think about it . . . a man reaching this particular point without realising it . . . the hopelessness about the future . . . then a young person is the very opposite — full of belief in the future. A relationship with a person like that takes care of the vacuum. It gives a validity to the future, so there is obviously a strong pull. Then you become tremendously dependant on that optimism of the other person if you are a man of the age of 40. The person's youth becomes absolutely, titanically important. It's ludicrous really because one is prepared to sacrifice everything that one had achieved materially or in one's work or whatever for a pretty lady who is young. Then you go through traumas and wreckage — which are perhaps quite titanic as they were with me — and then you meet someone else eventually but your marriage by then has broken up. Things get better in a way but perhaps you haven't been able to collect yourself together successfully into a perfect whole again because it's incredibly difficult to do so having been . . . bust wide open. It was a short-lived affair with the 25 year old woman. I don't treasure the memories of it at all. I look back on it as being a sickness really connected with a mental breakdown or the state of the male menopause.

I'm 48 and my wife is a bit older. There are four children — 6, 8, 16 and 20. I wouldn't say that the marriage was very good when I met the 25 year old lady — there were great holes in it, always had been — but there were other things to look to for fifteen to twenty years until the break came, and one did look to them because of the holes in the marriage. Nevertheless, there was a great companionship and affection in the marriage but one did very strongly turn to one's work because of the unsatisfactory relationship with one's wife; turn also towards other goals if they presented themselves — which would sweeten life — like buying things, setting up a garden or purchasing expensive cars. But they weren't enough in the end, when the 40's arrived, one had everything — and this is the tragedy of the male menopause that it comes when life should be at its sweetest. But it's then that a man feels there is nowhere to go, that there's no future except to continue in the same stale scene however well monied it might be, or satisfactory with regard to the reception one's work receives. Of course, one can, at that stage, manufacture challenges in one's work I suppose. I think I did because I started making a heavy investigation into a school of painting that dealt with the liberation of colour and changing my work pretty radically. Quite probably my work has been reinvigorated and revitalised by all that's happened. Certain complacencies do arise in one's work when one's got all the security one needs. After the male menopause situation, they disappear. The complacency may be something one longs to regain but it's not within one's grasp.

And the impact does not only affect the man. One of the things that always happens is that the wife suddenly starts trying to make herself more attractive — a reciprocal protest I suppose. My wife suddenly started dressing up — and my son told her she was making a fool of herself. She wanted me back although during the marriage she'd never allowed herself really to say that she loved me. She'd always baulked at expressing that. For some reason she'd never been able to express that, but, of course, when I was involved with the young lady, then she found that she did love me. She pursued me in all kinds of ways but at the same time felt enormously savage and once broke the young lady's room to pieces.

Then she went to Venice alone on a holiday and got involved with two very young Argentinian hustlers and an extraordinary scene took place then. Some sort of madness took over my wife then, although she wouldn't admit it. In apology I bought her a Morgan car and she took that to a little cottage by the sea — tearing around and living a very wild life . . . planning to spend £10,000 on a boat in which she was going away for two years to go round the world with these two men, one of whom was the age of her son, 19, and with whom she was having sex. That lasted for a few months. You see, the marriage had broken up. She had nowhere to go and no-one to do anything with. No way of breaking out herself. She's a good artist — a member of the Royal Academy — but not able to hang on to her work as I was. My work has always been much more important to me than hers to her. She did work a bit during the troubled times but she went off and did the same thing as I did. She ran after youth — a double scene in fact. By that time the whole thing had become so destructive that it hasn't healed yet. Wives of menopausal men retire into themselves.

Having gone through all that, I don't find younger women disturbingly attractive. Whereas, after the association with the young lady, all I could think of was young ladies. So I spent the next year and a half chasing after a broken love affair. But then the real breakage of the male menopause affected me and I started smashing up cars. I had accidents in two of my cars because of my state of mind. When I was smashing them up I am sure I was in a state and going through a period of insanity. It wasn't just getting into accidents — I was driving like a maniac, absolutely. I'm sure there was a subconscious death wish and at times I did think of suicidal inclinations.

There was quite a large amount of melancholia during these years and when I think back on the grip of the condition I think that to survive it is less likely than to endure it. But I talked to Ernie Wise the other day and he's just sailed through it. He hasn't had it and now he's 50 and you can see that he won't have it. But it caught and trapped me. And the defeating sense of staleness was with me before I met this young lady. It had to do with the responses and urgency of the situation. The needs and urges that one has at the time of the 40's obviously cause you to do things that you wouldn't have done ten years before. You might have met the same young lady and been enormously attracted, but, looking back, it was my advances that were desperate you might say. It then evolved into reciprocal love but I think if I'd met her at the age of 35 I wouldn't have felt the need to pursue the advances quite so strongly — I don't think it would have happened. When things get stale, in the early 40's or a bit later, if there's an opportunity, you start moving to some sort of self-destruction through another person. You sort of value your own situation and everything you've achieved as nothing compared with living with this person. And I'm sure that this happens to masses of men.

It's a diseased state and I'm still not fully healed, not out of the wreckage. If I apply the word melancholia to what happened it seems a very mild word because one was in a state of madness really for quite a long time. There were many times when I wished I could have talked things over with my wife having spent 20 years thinking in tune with her, thinking in union with her and planning everything that I did in conversations with her. We may not have been in love, but this relationship was very strong and I regret that it turned into such a savage thing. She liked having children. That was important to her and whatever resentment she had about me obviously faded as she accepted the marriage. She accepted it far, far deeper than I ever realised with regard to its comforts and luxuries; with regard to having pride in a husband although she didn't love him; and with regard to pride in her family. She referred to this pride at one time during the start of the break. I didn't realise it, but she was sinking into the marriage as if it was never going to stop — getting a sense of security. It had gone on a long time and it looked as if it would go on to the grave. So she was sinking into a state of inertia and when the marriage broke she couldn't do anything but stay put because over the years she'd sunk into the situation, believing in its indestructibility . . . as I had for that matter. Until finally she realised that it had broken and of course went right off course as I did . . . and now she will probably be bitter until she dies.

I attribute everything that's happened to the male menopause, and I tried to tell a psychiatrist once. My local GP referred me to him — he's a good chap and I spent one afternoon talking to him and afterwards he said a few words to my GP to the effect that I should go it alone. I think, at that time, I should have had more help . . . but it did take its own course and I've ended up in the situation that I'm in and I suppose that it could be worse — although it's still not right. I was given sleeping pills and tranquillisers but I didn't want to get involved with them — nor with drink. Although I did start turning to drink at one time — but that was no good either. The best thing was talking about it and getting other people to talk to me. Frank Muir insisted that I should call it involutional melancholia. He preferred that to the male menopause. And I've raised it with a lot of men of the right age who have been sitting for me: Ernie Wise, Tony Britton, Frank Muir. After talking to them all, I would say that some people avoid it, like some people tend to live to an old age. Some people get cancer and some don't. If it is metabolic it can affect some and not others. The female menopause affects women to a different degree so I wouldn't argue with the idea that some men don't seem to get it.

My solicitor has been through it. He felt his wife and family didn't need him any more so one day while they were on holiday he swam out to sea and just went on swimming and was going to die — but he heard his wife calling and so he swam back. He said this was very significant.

I remember trying to explain it to the young lady from the Royal College of Art. She greeted it with scorn. It was unacceptable to her because it dragged her down into a male menopause scene that prompted pretty violent attitudes against middle age and death in her eyes. She used to talk about the dead eyes of the tutors of the Royal College — scathing attitudes towards middle-aged people who represented a static and dead situation in life . . . and scathing about the fears of all of them for death. Now, in the married state before the smash I had all the normal feelings about lung cancer and all that. You smoke and then you think about it and you stop smoking and if you're driving a car you are as careful as possible because you might get crashed up — but that was as far as it went. I don't think I had particularly morbid fears of death . . . or dying.

Most of all what I feel now that I have come through a lot of it is a completely different person . . . re-invigorated, rejuvenated. I feel revitalised — restimulated. I certainly don't feel middle-aged. I don't feel those things I felt before the male menopause came along. It seems as if there is a period of rejuvenation that occurs after this strange experience — and you may be totally destroyed by the male menopause or you may come out of it revitalised, without the feelings of middle age that beset a person of about 40 or 45.

I don't know what the physiological facts are about this revitalising; but you do become at the age of about 40, 41, 42 . . . atrophied, and you don't know how to get out of it and so you think this is going to be your life for the rest of your life. And then, suddenly, you are torn to pieces by the male menopause and you come out of it, probably a mess still, but you're certainly not growing into a cabbage.

For almost every victim that we met, the menopausal problem seemed to be one of the differentials between the real and the apparent; the sought after and the achieved; the subjective and the objective; what the man was in the world outside and what he was in his head. Health, wealth, work, leisure: externally acclaimed success in all or any of these is not sufficient to bring immunity. Actual achievements (truly for some not very great) are not enough to ward off an attack. It is inside the heads of the victims that the causes are to be found. For some men, a simple cause of their secondary impotence might be hormonal imbalance — but secondary impotence is neither sufficient nor necessary . . . as symptom or cause. The male menopause is more complex and elusive than that.

We are of the opinion that the real significance of the male menopause is to be found in the standards of the victims' personal lives: first in their initial two years as babies; then in their adolescence; and finally when they come to accept that they are responsible, in particular and in general, for who and what they are and what is happening to them. The quality and quantity of their fantasies and aspirations in early life coupled with their ability to deal with reality factors, self-awareness and personal growth, at a later stage and their recognition of the consequent tensions and subtle implications will all govern their eligibility for the condition.

For such a candidate, the possibilities are not many: a mature realisation that he is in charge of almost everything but his death; surrender to despair; a song and dance act of loud peacock sexuality amplified in a mirror of vanity; self-deception and rationalisation that preach that old age comes as a welcome relief — early to those who deserve it; or a total Walter Mitty trip. Generally, for the menopausal male, the world becomes a jungle and he feels lost and alone — without the tools and weapons he needs for survival. For him reality is terrifying: time has caught up with him and tomorrow is today.

Today is the tomorrow he dreamed about yesterday . . . and all, far from being well, is a nightmare.

4 Renovation, Reparation or Preparation?

> There is no medicine for fear,
> Nor medication against death.

Many menopausal men rush to feeble palliatives. They try all kinds of remedies and recipes. They experiment with potions and pills — all in a desperate search for the universal panacea that will cure what they see as the cause of all their ills. As we have already described, those ills may vary from thinning hair and decaying teeth, failing eyesight and physical skills, slowing down of bodily and mental activity levels, waning sexual desire and performance, anxiety, depression . . . and so on. Their constant seeking tempts us to point out the likeness of misguided middle-age philosophers in their attempts to find the Elixir of Life.

Our men chase an equally unattainable product — a genuine revitalising Elixir of Youth. The fact that no such product exists does not prevent men in their thousands pouring enormous amounts of money into the hands of those commercial operators who con them into believing their pre-packed rejuvenators, pep-u-ups and erection creams and the like will do the job for them. Hairdressers, wig and hair-piece manufacturers and young men's outfitters all benefit similarly from the menopausal male in search of a costume and a disguise. Clothes, trendy glasses and discreet toupées — all these are dragged in to serve the cause of the dissembler and his need for camouflage. At best, these expensive props are inefficient, ineffectual and inefficacious . . . at worst, they draw attention to the condition that the menopausal man is trying to hide, thus broadcasting not only his unattractive situation, but also his pathetic and unintelligent way of handling it. Trichology, cosmetic surgery, pseudo-pharmaceutics and all the sartorial wizardry of the King's Road shine like beacons of hope in the foggy or kaleidoscopic world of our victims.

Health farms, yoga classes, meditation groups, massage salons, sauna baths and nudist clubs, all come in for their fair share of patronage. The combination of vaguely virtuous intentions, esoteric practices, disguised motives laced with a strong element of sexual frustration, make them suitable targets for the menopausal male. His search for revitalising diets, slimming treatments, bio-energetics exercises and health food rituals parallels his quest for a 'genuine' aphrodisiac and sex-aids 'that really work'. Sensitivity about going bald, lengthening eyesight, getting fat (usually euphemistically referred to as "putting on weight" in spite of the moral tale told by Wells in *The Truth About Pyecroft*), going grey, feeling grey, looking grey and fearing impotence drives men in their thousands into the arms of a thriving commercial set-up based on pandering to the inadequacies of menopausal men, and this is how they regularly come across to an attractive young woman hair-dresser who works in a smart, West End men's salon.

I'm sure that lots of secretaries will tell you that the first sign in their boss that he is going through this particular stage of life is that he will attempt a new hair-style and then progress — or regress if you like — into clothes and then younger ladies.

If they are going bald they will either resort to a toupee or have a perm or lighten it all up a bit. They have this thing that curls do tend to make them look younger. They may start by teasing their hair around the receding part of the hairline. Then they will go in for the 'break' instead of a parting so that the mingling of the lines camouflages the thinning. For a time this kind of treatment, together with the infamous combing forward, will suffice, but there comes a point when even they recognise that there is no hair there and then they will consider resorting to a toupee.

But none of them ever actually speaks out about what is happening or what they are trying to do — or have me do. Most of them will shun it completely. If I do ask any of them why they want their hair left longer they may say, "Well, I'm approaching 40 so I'm wanting to look a bit different," and a few may say they'd like to look younger. But on the whole they try to avoid it if at all possible. They don't want to recognise what's happening to them if they can help it.

You see, there are lots of men who will come in just to have their hair cut by an attractive young woman. All they may need — and some of them need nothing at all — is a little bit by the ears, but just because they are being chatted up by an attractive girl they don't mind paying £2, £5 or £10. Honestly, all they want is a lot of talk to make them feel young, to make them feel needed, for that half hour so they don't really mind how much it costs.

There must be thousands of young women playing the part of surrogate something-or-other to menopausal men. Many of them will have no idea of how they are being perceived by their bosses, clients, of "daddy's friends". The whole ritual can sometimes be played out without the victim giving himself away — even to himself. However, when it comes to making a visit to a trichologist or cosmetic surgeon, no such avenue of external deception is open to the victim. When he gets to such a stage he has to come out in the open. Ellsworth Laing, the consultant surgeon, is sympathetic towards menopausal men who seek plastic surgery:

I'm sure there is such a condition. The male menopause, seen from a work or a social point of view is a real and very definite entity as far as I am concerned. The men invariably feel that they are deteriorating and want to retain — or even regain — their youth. There is this real need to prove themselves and this is why from time immemorial men have taken younger mistresses.

There are men who over-react by wearing trendy clothes — as I do for example — and keep their hair long. They may even be obsessed by the flashy, powerful sports car image. Then there are the others who go inward and get depressed. But what is certain is that it affects all we men one way or another — and while you may respond to it in different ways, there is no getting away from the reality of it as an entity.

The men who come to me professionally for treatment — cosmetic surgery that is — are usually depressed and miserable. Often, they look much older than they are, and their jaw lines have sagged. The men who want face lifts usually have younger wives. I don't think the wives have nagged them to come but it's clear that they are concerned that they look too old in comparison with their wives or they are afraid of the wives being attracted to a younger looking man.

Some come for hair transplants and I'm not convinced they are awfully satisfactory. I don't have any absolute evidence but my suspicion is that they don't last. Clients who want this kind of treatment are, I think, generally sexually inadequate — or think they are, which usually boils down to the same thing — and they feel that having more hair will give them more sex appeal. As I said, I have doubts about this area — but the face lifts are very good in my opinion.

A view from a different side of the business-world that caters for, among others, victims of the condition comes from Richard Price, who, with his wife (a State Registered Nurse), runs a sex shop in Croydon under her maiden name of Phyllis Wright Health and Hygiene.

Quite a few of our customers, both men and women, do come in and complain about the male menopause as such. On average, we may get four to five men each day with problems to do with erections: either they can't get one at all or they lose it too quickly. And they come from all kinds of backgrounds. We have civil servants, postmen, builders and millionaires. Quite often what has happened is that their doctors have been generally unhelpful — just didn't want to know or had no idea what to do. Occasionally we get a customer who has been to an enlightened doctor who has put him on testosterone injections — but only too often they don't work so the man ends up here like all the others. We frequently also get men who have been on some drug like Valium or Librium and they have developed erection problems. Now, in that case we can help since coming off the drug and taking some of our vitamin E tablets can help enormously. It works wonders if the man is just stressed and strained.

In some cases the real problem lies with the wives. There are those men who have used their wives as receptacles for their penises and that's all. One woman said to me, "All he wants me for is sex. It makes me feel as if the only thing I can ever be is a vehicle for sex." Inevitably such wives become — sooner or later — unwilling partners. Then there are the men who have a low sex drive and the wife is the one who seems to be over demanding. But I suppose the most common and real crisis comes when the wife is inhibited or disinterested in the bedroom. As a man gets older he needs more and more positive stimulation from his wife. It takes more and more to turn him on and if his wife isn't interested and willing to work out what to do for him, then it's no good. We've had men in here actually begging us to help them change their wives' attitudes, but there's nothing we can do, apart from stressing the need for proper communication and perhaps suggest reading a good book which deals sensibly with sexual problems and behaviour.

Many men are helped by sexy magazines. Some say they are the only things that get them going. We sell them now. We used not to but so many men want them . . . and of course selling them helps to pay the rent.

Quite a lot of men try the Blakoe Energiser and in my experience it's by far the best thing for impotence. I reckon it helps as many as 70% — but it is expensive at nearly £10. Sometimes the men will say, "But my wife wouldn't like me to wear one of those," and I tell them they are no different from glasses and she doesn't mind them wearing those so where's the difference? There is a lot more resistance to them than there is to such things as 'sex-booster' tablets which do no more good than any dextrose you can get from the chemist.

When it comes to men who have wives younger than they are — perhaps by 15 years or more — we do get a lot of sad cases. They will say, "She wants more sex than I can give her so what can I do?" and this is where a prosthetic can be very useful . . . We had an architect of 65 who was having an affair with his 40 year old secretary. It saved the day so well when he couldn't get an erection that they are now happily married. Then there was an elderly man who was completely impotent. He came back after he'd bought one and he was so pleased, "At long last I can give her a bit of pleasure".

I'm sure that a prosthetic could often be the answer for a man with the menopause, although ideally, of course, one wants to cure the cause of the condition.

Some men turn to a prosthetic (be it hair, teeth or another vital part) but many more turn to alcohol. This form of retreat is well known, well documented and totally condoned by society — indeed encouraged — provided it is not overdone. Surgeon Vice Admiral Sir Dick Caldwell of the Medical Council on Alcoholism:

Possibly one of the many reasons why men between the ages of 40 and 45 start to drink too much is that very few of them actually get to the top. The great majority always visualise themselves attaining the position of boss of their department or head of something or other, but they have to accept, sooner or later, that they are going to be frustrated. When that time arrives, they will probably say, "Well, I remember when I was 30 I used to think I'd be manager of the bank. Now I'm 45 and I'm chief cashier . . . actually that's all I am and all I'm ever going to be," and when that occurs there is a despondency that overtakes them.

I know from my own experience: I used to be fond of a game of tennis, golf, any strenuous exercise, but you find in your late 40's that, whereas you used to be able to play two games of squash perfectly happily, now you feel rather tired after it. A sense of one's waning powers emerges — not necessarily sexually, because I don't think that does automatically happen as early as that, but a general sense of not being such a tough guy as you were in your late 30's. Then, immediately, an overall fear or anxiety can set in — and they certainly can cause impotence to occur.

If the man also turns to heavy drinking, as many do, his liver may become affected and it is fairly well established that if the liver begins to fail, a hormone imbalance is created and the man begins to develop secondary female characteristics. Breasts may begin to appear and the hair on his face and pubes may start to disappear — and his sex drive will certainly be affected, so impotence may then add to his other problems and the whole thing will become a downward spiral.

The suggestion that a man might begin to develop secondary female characteristics takes us straight into the whole area of mirror symptoms. While Dick Caldwell was putting over a very special point of view, related to definite physiological factors, we have met many men and women — lay people as well as medical authorities — who believe that the whole concept of the male menopause is based upon men mirroring what is happening. Indeed, more than one medical specialist has put the point to us that, in terms of human development, the woman is the model and the man a mere variation.

There are cases of men who, just like in *couvade* or other forms of sympathetic magic and rituals, experience themselves what is happening to their wives. They suffer regular monthly pains, depressions and temperature variations. They experience pregnancy sickness and whims as well as ante-natal anxieties and post-natal depressions. And male phantom pregnancies are not entirely unknown.

In addition, there is the more easily understood aspect of the man's over-response to the woman's own symptoms, whether menstrual or menopausal, and this indeed may be a powerful and common factor, whereas true 'mirror symptoms' are unusual. While it is perfectly understandable that a man should find it difficult to know how to deal with the irrational behaviour patterns that may be displayed by a menopausal woman, there is no sufficient and necessary cause to be found in her behaviour that will dictate that he himself will go male menopausal while trying to relate, help or just cope. It is more likely that if he over-responds it will reflect his laziness in dealing with the woman; his flight from her reality through a factitious defence mechanism; or his own hopeless inadequacy to face up to any sign that an ageing process is around and for real.

Approaching a doctor is not easy for many of the men who feel they are going down with the male menopause. Nor is it easy for them to find the right kind of doctor if they have sufficient courage to be able to approach one at all. For many the fear of mentioning impotence or mental illness is still all-consuming, since our social taboos are still so strong. If a man can get himself at least as far as a doctor's consulting room, it is tragic if he does not get the under-standing or perception he needs . . . and is entitled to. But unfortunately, many of our doctors are not equipped or interested enough to deal with problems of sexual activity; and, even more unfortunately, too many still view psychiatrists and psycho-therapists as being no better than witch doctors — who in their eyes are to be scorned. But before we get involved in things psychological, let us hear from a GP with a wider view than most. He is Dr Peter Scales, who from more than twenty years of general practice has had considerable experience of, and interest in this kind of problem.

Concerning the concept of such a thing as the male menopause, I would suggest that it is a complete misnomer. You cannot equate anything to the sexual difficulty which usually brings a male to my consulting room with a suggestion that he may be going through the menopause. You cannot equate it in any way with the female climacteric because even if the male's problem is hormonally based it involves quite a different section of hormones and a lot of difference in metabolism.

In any case, the testing for hormone ratios in the bloodstream is very, very difficult to get done. It is only undertaken in experimental centres in this country. I have had to work hard to get the appropriate departments to run testosterone studies as a routine check for patients with impotence — which is one of the symptoms, as I take it, for the so-called male menopause.

In my experience, the 'menopausal man' complains of a lack of erection ability or an inability to maintain an erection. This immediately puts his sexual prowess into question and he becomes disappointed and depressed. His partner may share this disappointment and depression — and a certain amount of disillusionment too. One of two things happens as a result of the impotence. They may become neurotic and the depressions may continue due to lack of strength, being run down, tired and miserable and all that, which will do nothing but reinforce the problem of the impotence. Or, they may decide to ignore the whole thing, discard their sexual life and live as brother and sister trying to make a relationship that way.

Whether the disuse of the sexual organs leads to an atrophy in the glandular structure and, therefore, a diminution in their output is very difficult to say. Personally, I don't think it occurs. I think it is purely an attitude of mind, associated with a very chronic mild depressive phase. I think the average story concerns a middle-aged male who has been married for twenty years give or take a bit. The marriage will have been successful as marriages go, but they will have got used to each other. The children will have grown up. They themselves will have slowed down, with their interests narrowing. They will have been thrown back upon themselves and they will feel that they know each other so well that there is no possibility of surprise in anything they do. The dynamism in their relationship will have gone and so they will have become rather disinterested and disinclined in sex and everything else in their relationship. They may have other interests and hobbies which absorb their time, their commitment and their emotions quite a lot and because their marriage is happy and contented, they don't want to look elsewhere. They accept that their stimulation of each other is diminishing and therefore their sexual activity diminishes. When the habit of a ritual sexual relationship is broken and lost, it is very difficult to regain it with the same partner.

A colleague of mine once remarked on this subject of mid-life diminution or secondary male impotence, "The best therapy would be the introduction of a change of partner." But you can't do that. People are not prepared to accept change. If they are happily married, they want to stay that way. They don't want the complications of rushing around and having affaires here and there just to prove that they are still sexually viable. Their relationships with their spouses and families are more important to them.

Most of my male patients over the age of 45 are likely to mention in a jocular fashion that they may be going through 'the change', but they don't believe it themselves. What they are really asking is why should they have suddenly become impotent. They are saying, "Why has this happened? What has gone wrong?" and are hoping that there will be something outside themselves that is to blame. This is why they mention the possibility of male menopause. Every one of us is loath to blame ourselves for something we do wrong. It is far more acceptable to our own psyche to find an external cause to blame. Then we don't have to consider the possibility that we have not given the matter sufficient thought or dealt with it properly. We don't wish to accept that kind of reason — we'd much rather blame something else. Therefore I get male patients with secondary impotence who put up this idea of the male menopause to explain everything. They have all their own reasons for invoking it.

A lot of them use it to rationalise their behaviour if they go on the rampage after young women. And a lot of them come to me when they have failed on that circuit. A typical example is the business executive in his 50's. He may have been at an office party and had an interesting experience with a 28 year old secretary. When he tried to follow it through he was horrified to discover his incapacity to function sexually with her according to his own expectation or to her needs. He may still be sleeping with his wife or he may not have had erections for some time. But nine times out of ten he will have given up his sexual relationship with his wife, but not his interest in sex. The chances are that both he and his wife have lost interest in sexual activity with each other through boredom and this opportunity at the party revives him enough to make advances. Then he gets into bed and finds to his horror that he can't get an erection. This is one of the commonest occurrences possible and an enormous amount of my patients have this kind of problem. I believe that the media is responsible for a great deal in this area since they publish the idea that not only should one jump into bed immediately with someone fresh but that when you do there will be an explosive capacity and everyone will be swamped with multiple orgasms.

Let's face it, this just doesn't happen. An older man's first sexual experience with a new partner for many years will often end up in disaster for the man. But if it is persisted in and he has an understanding approach from the partner he has chosen, if he is interested enough and if he has been perfectly normal in the past, then he will rapidly get back his prowess at any age. It is important that he should have an understanding partner though. The last thing a man wants in such a situation is an aggressive woman. That will frighten him off more than enything and he will entirely shut off. The woman needs to be able to examine the problem in a neutral fashion to start off with and get the man to talk about the situation. Very often, merely by talking about it, he will get interested in it and the sexual implications and one thing will lead to another . . . and he will be away.

It is possible that the so-called male menopausal crisis can be dealt with in the family itself. It is important that the wife should examine herself as well as her husband. She should ask herself if there is anything in her past that is *supposed to be buried* that could bring out more of her innate sensuality. She should see if she could stimulate it more because by doing so she would stimulate herself . . . and also her partner. It is quite surprising how much information about themselves partners keep from one another. A couple came to me because their sex life had gone into a state of decay and the husband appeared to be totally and utterly impotent. They were supposed to have tried everything including talking about it at great length, but he was still incapable of achieving an erection. They came to me for counselling and there seemed to be nothing in their histories to point to any causation until I came to the end of my enquiries when I asked, as I always do, if there was any question of fetish objects. Eventually he admitted that he had a rubber and plastic fetish. At first the wife found it difficult to accept when I explained it to her. But later, when she found that the mere purchase of a plastic mac — and wearing that alone — produced an astounding effect, she was more than ready to understand, and comply. Her husband became far more virile than he had been at any time previously in the marriage. Tragically, too many cases like this get passed over when couples could be helped. In the case of any man who suggests that he might be menopausal I would suggest that the wife should broach the subject of sex fetishes. It can never do any harm.

The area we are considering is filled with businessmen of the executive type and they suffer, *par excellence*, from secondary impotence. Firstly because their business drives tend to overshadow their sex drive if it has been on the lowish side. Secondly, and very often, because they have risen from a moderate background and their wives, who came from that same background, have not risen with them and are no longer to be seen as desirable sex objects. I read an article in *Playboy* recently that advocated a new marriage every five years to cope with this kind of problem — and others due to the fall-off from boredom after five years or so. Clearly, though, this is impractical and, in any case, when you have a good relationship with somebody you want to keep it. I certainly try to support relationships as long as I can. If they cannot rejuvenate their sex life I would try to help them come to terms with the situation and make the best of the good side of their relationship. Why not? They have, say twenty years of a good marriage between them; they have built it together; they now have things in common — a family, grandchildren, happy memories and all that kind of thing. So why not keep them? And at the same time, of course, continue the counselling if there is the slightest glimmer of hope.

I can only think that the phrase male menopause came about because some women mistakenly thought their menopause meant the approaching twilight of their sexual lives. So, when a period of impotence overtook a man, the same logic worked in reverse and the connotation was given to men.

Peter Scales stresses — quite rightly in our opinion — the importance of counselling when dealing with conditions similar to the male menopause, and while we find ourselves in disagreement with him in equating the "so-called male menopause" with secondary impotence, we respect his view that the phrase is not only a misnomer, but is also based upon a false assessment of what happens during the female menopause. We also applaud his implied recommendations that anyone who is to help in these circumstances must tackle the problem in the manner of peeling an onion. The only solution is for the man himself to be able to see into the layers of his psyche and perceive what has gone wrong. Awareness itself, as Fritz Perls said, is therapeutic — and there are those who believe very strongly that wise counsel from other people, lay or professional, can help the victim to achieve this sense of awareness. We shall shortly be presenting the views of three professionals who are of this view.

Certainly, a state of mental and emotional upheaval is symptomatic of the male in menopause. For example, we have come across a number of cases who seemed to fit the archetypal pattern as if it had been made for them, and their situation regarding 'purpose in life' was so ambivalent and vacillating that in the end they abdicated from the struggle completely and compensated for any early maternal deprivation they might have suffered by rushing into the arms of Mother Church. Some went no further than embracing, somewhat over-enthusiastically, a 'new' religion, but others — a very definite fringe minority, in a state of real instability — actually took holy orders. No doubt they would be aghast at our judgement that sees their escape route as no better than that of the man who rushes around applying for jobs or the man who validates his image by pinching the bottoms of young girls. They are all feeble efforts: the girl-seekers are saying, 'Please tell me that I am here' and the religion-seekers are saying, 'Please tell me what to do now that I am here'.

When a man is in such a state of emotional chaos he is easy prey for false gurus, immodest prophets and quasi-therapists of the 'psycho/hypno' variety. This is not the place to conduct an exposé of these individuals but it is relevant to observe that many of them come into their financial own when dealing with a menopausal male who is an outstanding case for the fleecing treatment since he is already mutton dressed as lamb . . . and as such a lamb he often goes without a murmur to the slaughter — not even the whimper that Eliot gives to the way the world ends. But when men get to a stage where their jealousy and envy, bitterness and resentment, can be directed wholly without reason at their wives and families (as well as the world at large) and, often especially, at their sons, it is not unexpected that they will be seen as targets for exploitation. When a man is in such psychological straits he draws attention to his vulnerability and broadcasts his weakness so loudly that he attracts the attention of the manipulators. Because of his lack of confidence generally, sapped even more by his sense of shame about what he is doing, he is also quite unable to take steps to gain redress or recompense even when he does discover that the 'therapy' he was being offered was a complete waste of his money.

But it is important that he — or perhaps at first his family — should have the benefit of skilled opinion and advice regarding the therapeutic steps he must take to get himself out of his unhappy state. It is highly desirable that everyone concerned should try to prevent him seeing his situation as a medical problem — with the exception of a minority as small as 1-2%, he will not be the victim of any organic dysfunction, hormonal or otherwise. It is one of the hazards of having a state medical system that too many of us are encouraged to interpret what are essentially personal and social problems of inter-action as medical problems — and a terrifying sign of this is the growing dependence of millions of people on the far too freely prescribed anti-depressants and tranquillisers. Des Rayner is only one among thousands of men whose condition has been made worse by dispensations of librium and valium, etc.

What is really needed is a sense of proportion in all concerned, since the menopausal man's most notable deficiency is precisely in this area. Retaining, regaining or creating this sense of proportion must be one of the menopausal man's first goals . . . Cleobulos, King of Rhodes, (c. 630-559BC) described it as keeping the golden mean, and while our victim might need to discover areas where he can rediscover euphoria, with regard to his vision of himself he can follow no better advice.

> Man is his own star, and the soul that can
> Render an honest and a perfect man
> Commands all light, all influence, all fate.

Earlier we implied that an obsession with freaky diets and eating habits was not to be encouraged as a way of coping with the menopausal condition. This we stand by, but also recognise that a proper reappraisal of attitudes to food and drink may be a good starting point for the middle-aged man who is struck down, if only in his own eyes. Biologically, we are what we eat and drink; psychologically we are what we do and say. Thus, it is of the greatest importance that any man who feels he is, or is about to become, a menopausal victim should come to understand, accept and act upon the fact that we all really do control our own destinies and that there is little point in blaming other people, things or events for what we have or have not accomplished. The sins of commission and omission are our own sins — and we try to opt out of that responsibility at our peril.

This is how Ron Geesin, ('composer for all media and supplier of notions'), puts it in his book of poems *Fallables:*

OPENING FOR GOING THROUGH

If one is not true to
and fails to realise
one's expressive possibilities
one is liable to be legally sued by oneself
for misrepresentation.

We have already suggested that vanity is quite out of place as an attitude to living and will bring nothing but psychic poverty in the long run. Vanity, not pride, is what Prince Lucifer might properly have been accused of. Vanity is the sin that goes before the fall. Pride is the responsibility of each human being for what happens to each and all of us and is one of the most admirable and important of all human attributes. Proper pride motivates purposeful actions that improve the status of all of us — not only the protagonist — and gives us that strength that enables us to take hold of our lives. In *Julius Ceasar,* Shakespeare puts it this way:

There is a tide in the affairs of men,
Which, taken at the flood, leads on to fortune;
Omitted, all the voyage of their life
Is bound in shallows and in miseries.
On such a full sea are we now afloat,
And we must take the current when it serves,
Or lose our ventures.

Men at some time are masters of their fates;
The fault, dear Brutus, is not in our stars,
But in ourselves, that we are underlings.

Someone once said that the real poets of the 20th Century are the psychologists. Our first contributor from that area is Dr Robert Sharpe, founder of The Institute of Behaviour Therapy and himself in private practice in Wimpole Street.

When you consider information like that contained in the 1944 paper (*The Male Climacteric,* Heller and Myers, see Appendix C) you must consider fads and fancies in the field. Things come and go. The thing of the 60's was the fantastic female orgasm. It made life unbearable for vast amounts of the population who were all doing it anyway and enjoying themselves. But it made them sit up and think, "Goodness me, am I missing out?" The fads of topicality must not be overlooked or over-rated. This paper could have spiralled off into a whole battery of research which said, "NO, men don't" or "YES, men do", but it didn't. In any case, papers aren't really taken very seriously as having contributed something concrete until at least one other faction with no axe to grind has reproduced the same results. So, until I am given the straightforward evidence that men at age X don't produce so much testosterone or there is some sort of hormone imbalance, the idea of the male menopause is meaningless to me. I can't use the term. I can't work with it. And even if someone proved that it occurred I would say, "OK, I'll work in conjunction with a medic who restores the hormone balance or whatever, while I'm *still* working at the environmental level."

This is because I'm a behaviour therapist and see my client as an on-going inter-action with his environment. It is therefore meaningless for me to know that a person is phobic. I need to know (a) the sort of responses he makes and (b) the configurations of situations in the environment which spark him off. Similarly, it's not very much use to me to know that a man may or may not be under-going the male climacteric. I would need to know, as I would with a woman at the so-called change of life, how that internal change impinges on the environment and what the environment does back.

Let's look at some of the factors. Women quite clearly do have physiological changes. They stop periods and they have hormonal changes. Now we're programmed in our society to accept that if a person changes physically they might also change psychologically. If you break your arm, you're expected to be a bit crotchety — so it is accepted that you might appear a bit under the weather, ill or what have you. We are programmed that way. But many so-called primitive societies don't notice a damned thing at the climacteric. The woman stops bleeding and that's all. In other words, there is a large expectancy problem. It's just like pain in childbirth: women expect to feel pain — so they do. In other cultures where women don't expect it they don't feel it. Pain is a very curious psycho-physiological phenomenon. You can gash yourself very badly in the heat of a rugby match and not notice a thing. But if you do the same thing in cold blood it will hurt like hell. This is the expectancy problem, and with so much scientific knowledge brought to bear upon women's climacteric, they are expected to go through behavioural changes. A man isn't expected to. Nothing demonstrable alters in a man. He doesn't stop bleeding because he's never bled in the first place and so on. So, one of the reasons why we don't see a male climacteric problem may be that we don't expect to see it — which is not to say that it does not occur.

Certainly in clinical practice one sees in the mid-40's age group a large number of people who expect to start functioning at a lower level. They say, "Oh well, I'm in my 40's now . . . what do you expect from somebody that age?" It would be interesting to know how much that is a product of simply comparing themselves with younger blood and how much a product of internal change. How much it was a matter of expecting not to function so well and how much due to hormonal change. You see, different things are expected of you when you're in your 40's from when you're in your 20's or 30's. For the majority of people, the expectations of the 40's are that they will be giving way to a growing family — young people who will be very active. They will be at the fairly arbitrary age of thinking about winding down in work, stopping being all that productive. The man will be inter-acting with a woman who is changing and expecting to change from a behavioural point of view. And here a certain amount of modelling will take place. We know that people learn vicariously from watching other people and if one member of a family sees another exhibiting quite clear changes of behaviour, they may rub off. This is to be seen dramatically in men who literally blow up and have phantom pregnancies to accompany their wives.

At this time in life, the man will not be as strong as he was. Nor will he be as quick. Billions of brain cells will have died by this time. One might ask, "Why didn't he have his climacteric earlier since billions of brain cells will have died between ages 20 and 30?" and the answer lies in the fact that for all individuals sources of stress combine in an additive manner. For example, a phobic person may also have marital and financial difficulties. If one day a letter arrives from the bank manager and the wife starts creating at the breakfast table, those two environmental factors will produce a level of stress that will cause the old phobia to resurge again. The same process obtains with the middle-aged busy executive who might be able to cope with the very high level of stress coming from a heavy work-load day after day — but when his car breaks down, or he is involved in an accident or some other stress comes along to take him beyond his level of optimal stress, then his behaviour might start to disintegrate. (Incidentally, if he went below his optimal stress level his behaviour would similarly disintegrate because he wouldn't be keyed up enough.) So, taking the case of the man with the change of life problem, he may well cope with the younger guys coming along at work so that he doesn't get the more taxing jobs; he may cope with his kids growing up and making more demands — becoming more independent beings and possibly rivalling him; but when his wife has a bad time in her menopause and sexual activity drops off and inter-personal relationships in the house get a bit twitchy, this adds yet another slice of stress and may be the straw that breaks the camel's back. His anxiety level, which has been manageable before, soars to a degree where the person becomes totally terrified, and he suffers a behavioural disturbance which is attributed to the male menopause. This is why it's very important to me not just to give them labels.

It's relatively meaningless to me to hear the term menopause, whether it's male or female. I want to know about the environmental factors so that I can start dealing with the stress areas individually. So, if sex relations have broken down, let's do some marital therapy. If he has become downtrodden at work and everybody is walking over him and getting promoted over his head, let's teach him how to be more assertive. I wouldn't address myself to the diagnostic label at all. In fact, I find it if anything misleading since, even if you assume it exists, what do you do about it? You can't chop it out and you can't give it a drug. There's nothing you can do with it since it is merely a descriptive term. Now the functional or behavioural analysis will tell me how the man — with or without his climacteric — is getting on with his environment. That I can watch, that I can measure. And if he has lost his self-image or even left work I can gradually get him to be more assertive at work or teach him how to get started on getting interviews again. I can lead him to a situation where he can go to the boss's office and say, "Excuse me, but I am rather fed up with the hum-drum stuff I'm getting. Can I have a change of tack?"

If the problem seems to have been initiated in the family environment I would get the whole family involved and have a council of war . . . hopefully, perhaps a council of peace. We would get down to discussing and describing what was going on. I would certainly bring in the kids because they are usually very insightful and often worried about the situation so they would actually welcome the chance of having some advice on making dad feel a bit more wanted. I would certainly try to help them understand the principles of empathetic listening — active listening that says, "I understand how you feel. I'm feeling it with you." It's the kind of listening that a good therapist does with his client.

If the problem seemed to centre on the man dressing too young so that it was an embarrassment, I would draw his attention to it and try to get him to understand that it was one way of fighting feelings of anxiety and growing old. Having established that, I would try to work on his anxieties via a different route. I would also be prepared to line up his wife, family, friends and workmates — learned opinion in fact — to substantiate that he looked daft in his inappropriate gear. I would also reinforce the good behaviours of his that went along with his 'cloak of youth'. If he played a good game of squash at 45 I would want that to be maintained. It would be a matter of fading out what was inappropriate so that he was a bloody good, active 45, not a 'quite-clearly-mutton-dressed-up-as-lamb-45'.

The most complicated problem is when the man gets himself into the young bird thing. One needs to know what he wants from young women that he's not getting — and is there any hope that his wife can provide it. If it's nice firm boobs and chronological age 20, his wife will not be able to help — and then one must ask what does he want those things for anyway. But it is virtually never the case that a person's set of requirements cannot be replaced by others and it may be that he is chasing young birds because his wife is nagging. OK, he may like the thrill of the chase but if his wife could give him a more reasonable life — which she could manage by learning how to emit non-nagging behaviour — then he might no longer have the need to career around after young bits of skirt.

My framework of learning principles says that all problems have been learned and the therapy consists of learning how not to have a problem. I am sure that most of the cases that could be described as male menopausal would be more than suitable for such a process — and that means ten to twenty sessions of individual or group work, not years of analysis. It gets them moving in the right direction again . . . and then life takes over.

Our next contribution comes from Dr Michael Bott who is a consultant psychiatrist on the staff of a South Coast mental hospital.

It seems sensible to look at the menopause syndrome as an entity — affecting both men and women and probably having similar causation in both sexes. I would describe what occurs as involutional melancholia — corresponding to the depression that sets in with people who come unstuck with the menopause.

I think it is appropriate to look at both men and women because of the differentials that surround the menopause in women themselves. There is real separation between the cessation of menstrual activity and emotional disturbances: they are not necessarily synchronous, nor do they necessarily occur in the same people. The variations are similar to those surrounding menstrual and pre-menstrual depression and those differences are highly correlated with personality. The sort of dramatic changes that one sees in some menopausal women are much more common in the neurotic type who is sensitive emotionally — and I think this also applies to victims of the male menopause. The chances are that they will have exhibited some form of personality abnormality long before things go wrong menopausally.

I would expect that many of the men who see themselves as having fallen victim to the male menopause would have a history that makes it quite predictable. People are seldom very experimental in how they behave. They don't go into a situation with an open mind or with a relatively small number of ideas about what might happen and then find out. They go in with convictions — and convictions are straitjackets that will determine behaviour, since the way we behave depends to a great extent upon how we feel at the time . . . and, more importantly, how we expect to feel once we are in the situation. This brings up one of the big problems in terms of treating impotence — one of the regularly apparent symptoms of the male menopause. The men expect that when they attempt any sexual activity that it won't work — and so they are pre-ordained. And in the wider context of those victims who are thrashing about, trying to find some new meaning, trying to sort themselves out — they are doomed from the beginning since they are using all the old strategies from the past, and ones that have failed them constantly, to try to find new ones. And of course it doesn't work. They are relying on their previous suppliers of ego-boost yet knowing that they are going to fail and not deliver the goods. They are, in all probability, unaware that they need to find it in themselves and quite incapable of changing the old suppliers. To over-simplify considerably, they can't achieve maturity. Their personal philosophy does not help them to deal with the question of their own mortality: they can't come to terms with the question of their personal death.

If a man has been used to getting validation of himself from other people and has relied on his physical appearance to help — or even to do it for him — then he has placed himself in a position over which he has only limited control at best. However, if he had relied on what he said and how he acted he would have had much more control. Those factors would not inevitably change so much as he aged. There is no doubt that depression sets in if the validation one has been getting from performance in life or work evaporates — and one isn't able to replace it with other sources.

The case of the writer (p.105) is a good example of a man who has actually done something about it. He has come to terms with it and changed his set of ideals. He saw that it had all gone wrong and fallen apart so he sat back and said, "This is non-viable as a system. Let's re-think it." And he did precisely that in a way that makes sense. Now that's nice — and it surely must be encouraging to all the others. But the change must be purposeful. There's no point in flailing about making changes for the sake of change — and even less if the changes are no more than old friends in new clothes. Take the case of men leaving their wives for younger women. I have two patients myself who are interesting contrasts and they help make the point. The first is similar to the man described on p.71. He has taken off at age 50 with a bird of 25. He is totally besotted with this girl. He can't face age; he is obsessed with remaining young, can't bear people to know his age, dresses young and wears a toupee — the whole lot. He's leaving a wife I think of as an attractive woman and entirely appropriate for him. Interestingly enough, his wife had been frigid for a time but when that cleared up the threat of her mature sexuality was too much for him and he had to take off into youth again — or so he thought.

The second case is quite different in cause although similar in effect. The man in this case came to see me because, in brief, his wife and family thought he had gone completely nutty. He was a man in his early 50's and he had met a young woman who shared his tastes and he was giving up the family home and everything else to go and live with her. Previously he had been faithful to his wife and for years and years a model parent but suddenly it all blew up. Of course, his wife and family thought he must be mad to give up his beautiful home and lovely family etc. to take up with this woman. But after talking with him for a long time, I came to the conclusion that he was making the decision on absolutely the right sort of basis. The girl wasn't a sex bomb or a symbol of youth. She was something of a personality bomb but she met his real needs as well. He told me he was happier than he had ever been in his life. As far as I could see he was completely and utterly sane. He was making the right decision at the right time — and was totally non-menopausal.

Certainly, mid-life is a time of questioning and saying, "Where am I? What have I done with my life?" and one of the most important questions is, "What sort of marriage do I have?" I would suggest that if one is going to categorise people who might be specially at risk regarding the menopause, I would put forward people who are in bad marriages — and the conclusion one draws is that if you're going to query your marriage and say, "What is its quality?" one ought to do it before you get to mid-life.

In fact there ought to be a continual reviewing process so that people don't wait until they get to mid-life to ask these questions — to decide if life is giving them what they want. The alternative gives you a bloke who wanders through life without wondering what he's up to. He can too easily find himself in mid-life in the wrong job, married to the wrong woman and bloody fed up with all of it — and then you have a classic case for menopausal explosion. Whereas a man who is reviewing his life periodically will be able to see that he is not going to be managing director of the firm and can say, "OK, in that case I won't work so hard. I won't bother so much in those directions. I'll diversify into other activities." He is much more likely to avoid a dramatic crisis and may sail through the menopause without noticing it.

There are other things that undoubtedly predispose to catastrophes at this time of life. One of them is being an obsessional; if you are, and you haven't been able to do anything about it during your 20's or 30's you are almost certainly going to come unstuck later on. It works like this: obsessionals have behaviour patterns that are rigidly organised and don't relate to the circumstances. They usually have high standards and are meticulous in everything — in entirely inappropriate ways. Classically, you have a man who is accustomed to doing it all himself, running the firm, doing his business, whatever it may be. He is very bad at delegating — claiming that nobody else can do it as well as he can. "It's pointless to delegate . . . they will only make a mess of it and I shall have to put it right." So he overloads himself with work and finally he crashes because he simply can't keep up. He can't work such long hours, physically he's not so strong, his memory begins to go a bit . . . and he becomes a dead ringer for a menopausal crisis.

Another important predisposing factor is one I touched on earlier — a dependance upon non-controllable sources of personal validation. If you are going to depend upon other people's reactions to you, to tell you that you're a good guy, then you haven't got a stable input. You will be in a much safer situation if you can ensure that you gain part of your validation yourself — achieving it from a sense of satisfaction with your own excellence and not depending so much upon other people. The chances are therefore, to over-simplify again, that people with menopausal crises are likely to be extroverts rather than introverts. Extroverts get their boosts by getting high on people so there is a concern with relationships and personal appearance. Introverts tend to be self-boosting and do not have the same concern with their inputs. The extrovert male in mid-life ought therefore to give some thought to being slightly less extroverted, to having some internal personal interests and so having at least some control over what is happening to him and not relying exclusively upon the environment and his inter-action with it.

Generally, therefore, the people who get caught by menopausal crises need some help to look at themselves as individuals, to analyse where they are in a personal sense, to assess how they fit into life, and to understand how they can balance their books better in the future. And this is something they don't need to take to a psychiatrist. OK, a psychiatrist may qualify as the right sort of person, but there aren't sufficient to go around. They need a sympathetic, intelligent person they can sit down and talk to — and here it is very much a matter of luck if they happen to know a sensible, sensitive person at the time when they need one. Certainly they are better off looking for that kind of help than rushing to their GP with a tale of impotence and asking for hormone replacement therapy.

It's too easy to suggest that hormonal changes are responsible for this mid-life crisis — especially the impotence. It's surprising how rarely one finds that impotent males have any disturbance of their hormonal levels, and I know of no research that suggests that it is the case with the male menopause. I am treating a man at the moment who is impotent. He doesn't have any sexual ideas. He doesn't masturbate. He doesn't get erections. Yet, to my amazement, his serum testosterone level was quite normal. I was convinced he had all the symptoms that would make him a good candidate and, without the test, it would have been only too easy to say, "Ah, yes, you don't do this or that, etc. We'll give you massive hormone pills." But that would have done no good at all. It would probably have made him feel ten times worse when nothing happened.

If some research were to establish a correlation between low hormone levels and the occurrence of these symptoms I would then be prepared to look at the possibility of the male menopause being a biological entity. In the absense of any such reliable data, I think it is a totally psychological entity.

It would seem pretty clear at this stage that the first task in front of any candidate for the male menopause — or for those who are trying to relate to him — is to learn to differentiate between symptoms and causes, and this is probably one of the most difficult tasks since the condition itself requires the confusion before it can exist. So the first step towards recovery must be for the man, and those who care for him, to do away with all dissembling, deceptions of self and others, and all forms of lies — no matter how white and how well intentioned in terms of 'protecting' feelings.

The man may not be able to achieve this in one step since he will probably have behind him a life of emotional hibernation and double-think, but at least his family and friends can do their uttermost to offer him a proper example, in the way they treat their own thoughts and feelings and one another's, as well as the man's. It would indeed be unfortunate if he were able to claim with any justification that they were 'picking' on him. It must be clear and incontrovertible that this new honesty applies even more to them than it does to him. He will be starting a long journey towards self-awareness and trying to get accustomed to change, and after a long history of personal non-growth and psychological under-development he will find the journey arduous and painful — and it will be some time before the therapeutic effects begin to accelerate and the pendulum begins to swing in his favour in a way that helps him feel good. After all, if he is to contemplate some drastic changes, the chances are that he will make plenty of drastic errors which will cause him grief. As Sydney Wasserman pointed out, he will need time. He may very quickly begin to feel good about facing in a new direction, but that will not protect him from the hurt he must experience as a realisation of past waste dawns upon him — and neither should it, if he is to achieve a complete recovery. As the psychiatrist, Reilly, in Eliot's *Cocktail Party* puts it:

> Your business is not to clear your conscience
> But to learn how to bear the burdens of your conscience.
> . . . some men have to learn much worse things
> About themselves, and learn them later
> When it's harder to recover, and make a new beginning.

Adjusting to reality and taking life and other people — as well as himself — for what they really are, will not be achieved overnight for such a man. It will require consummate effort on his part and an understanding from others that he will need a tremendous amount of psychological self-space if he is to manoeuvre freely enough to find himself, other people and the quality of his relationships with them.

Peeling off the masks to find the psyche beneath the skin can be a painful process. What everybody must realise is that it is painful enough for the man to do it himself, but once others get their fingers behind his psychic contraceptive membrane and start to pull, the pain will in all probability be too much for him to take. He will, in very truth, 'lose face'. His real hope is to learn how to discard his masks by and for himself and he will then experience the skin-shedding process as an act of discovery, of self-revelation, of self-disclosure — and not one of exposure.

Re-orientation and re-definition of life styles is much easier when you have not invested a life-time's energy into pursuing what is shown to be a goal 180 degrees away from the new objectives. It is not easy to drop well-established habits of chauvinism, sexism, sexual snobbery and a generally superficial attitude to the world, the flesh and the Devil-Joneses. Nor is it palatable to look upon, say, twenty five years of psychological, emotional, intellectual, physical and perhaps even financial investment only to discover that all the banks were bankrupt at the beginning.

Perhaps one of the most difficult lessons for the menopausal male to learn is that his spiritual income is more essential to him than any of the acquisitive rewards of the rat race to affluence. After years of racing, it is hard to accept, at first and in toto, that the Human Race should not be a race at all. After years of competing, it is not easy to see that life is not a competition . . . or, for those who make it into one, the only prize they will ever win is an empty death after a pointless life. In an acquisitive, competitive society it takes courage and effort to co-operation and sharing as a way of life. There are only too many people ready and eager to convince everybody that everybody else is waiting to make a killing or pull off a rip-off. It is their only way to defend their own modus vivendi — and the menopausal male who succeeds in his attempts at radical change represents a threat and an indictment. They will not be among those who will be of any encouragement to him in learning that the essence of living lies in knowing when you need help and being able to ask for it in a way that will actually bring it from other people. The rat-race artists cannot consent to such a philosophy since it means they would have to be prepared to give from time to time — and acquisitive affluence depends upon a genius for taking, taking, taking.

The menopausal man needs to understand that security does not lie in the security boxes of the finance houses and that life's only reality is living and is not to be found in real estate. Man can only hope for two securities: the first is his own ontological security in himself as a person — and this is not easy to find — and the second is in the sure and certain security of his own death — and this is not easy to contemplate. Coming to terms with the death of his past will be a large step in preparation for accepting the inevitability of the future death of himself.

'Life begins at 40' is a well-known phrase. But in reality it begins *when* it begins — but there is no need for it to end at 40, menopause or no menopause. Birth happens to us all only once, but rebirth can occur again and again throughout life. Seen in such a light, the menopause comes as a cross-roads, not as a lay-by or dead-end. The options are chalked up and the menopausal man can choose. Our next contribution is from Dr James Hemming, psychologist, author and broadcaster, and this is what he has to say on the concept of the male menopause, and how to cope with it.

Some women have to put up with a lot during their menopause. It can be a time of considerable physical disturbance as well as emotional stress. To say the least, the hormonal balance, once upset, takes time to settle down again. But many women, apart from a moan or two about 'these damn flushes!' sail through the menopause without much trouble. It may be that these are the lucky ones whose bodies adjust easily, but it probably also helps if they start off well-adjusted and have a good perspective on life and themselves. It's when a life has not been very well fulfilled — when there has been a lot more frustration than satisfaction — that the menopause can hit hard. It is as though deep inside there is the gloomy feeling: 'Life has passed me by.'

All this applies to men also, to some extent. Men are spared the comparatively sudden menopausal switch from fertility to infertility in physical terms; the decline in their virility is more gradual. But a time arrives, nevertheless, when a diminution in the energies of youth, sexual and otherwise, can no longer be ignored. Consequently, life may, quite suddenly, begin to seem humdrum, meaningless, going nowhere. When this happens, the individual is faced with the need for a veritable 'change of life'. We might define the male menopause as the period between an acute sense of being threatened by the passage of the years and the attainment of a viable adjustment to the prospect of growing old. As is the case with women, the menopausal transition can be acute or long-drawn-out; it may be profoundly disturbing or hardly felt. The point is that, in one form or another, it happens and has to be dealt with. And how the crisis is dealt with depends, to no small extent, on previous experience and style of life.

It follows that, when this critical period arrives in a man's life, reactions to it vary, but some sort of snatching for reassurance is likely, the attempt to prove, 'I'm as good as ever I was'. This may take the form of chasing young women. At a time when a man feels his youth and potency are slipping away from him, a compulsion to demonstrate his virility anew can be strong.

Of course men of all ages are, and ought to be, interested in, and affected by, young women. That's natural. It is when you get a sudden explosion of such interest in a middle-aged man that you may well have a symptom of the male menopause. A man in this situation may feel driven to catch up on lost time before it is too late. This may be the outcome of an excessive conformity earlier on. The man may have been inclined to deny his natural impulses any expression, assuring himself that he was not the type to be interested in young women: 'I am married to a good woman who has given me two splendid children, therefore I am a respectable husband and father and I am going to stay that way.' That is, of course, an honourable and worthy position to take up, but it may have involved the guilty repression of feelings that are perfectly natural.

Feelings not allowed or accepted into full consciousness tend to kick back sooner or later, as we often see in the break-out of ex-convent girls. Add together anxiety about advancing years and residues of repressed sexually-toned feelings and you may end up with a bottom-spanking person or an ageing bank manager who goes fawning round the secretaries over-much at the office party, or elderly gentlemen who feel the need to pursue pretty girls in the park instead of resting content with a little discreet ogling.

These people are all expressing the same anxiety in different ways. They are, as it were, saying to every attractive young woman they meet: 'Here I am — a man. There are you — a woman. *Please* acknowledge my masculinity.' They may even be trying, belatedly, to live their unlived adolescence and youth. The result is not a potential relationship but a masquerade. Such compensatory behaviour is always sadly unrealistic, and defeats its own ends because it leads to rejection.

There are, of course, many examples of deep, genuine, and mutually satisfying relationships between older men and young women. For many men of any age — especially creative men — the young woman symbolizes something tremendously significant and is a vitalizing element in their lives and work. But this sense of relationship is deeply personal, relaxed and natural, and not a compulsion. It is the artificiality and impersonality of the bottom-spanking syndrome that makes it defective. No depth of relationship is present for either partner. The man's reaction is furtive and compulsive. It is the element of compulsion suddenly becoming obtrusive that is menopausal.

However, the upsurge of sexual interest is only one aspect of the menopausal syndrome. It is part of the middle-aged man's overall fear of losing grip. This makes him eager to prove to himself that, although he may be 40, or 50, or whatever, he is still an effective and significant person. This may link up with a sense of having lost out in the life stakes. He finds that he is not living up to his earlier dreams and hopes — life has failed to hand him the deal he expected. So he feels: 'For heaven's sake, I must do something. I can't settle for being a failure. I must prove that everything is still going for me.' He wants to feel that his dreams can still be attained, even though time is passing dreadfully fast.

Actually, such a man may have accomplished a great deal, but the sense of time running out gives him a disturbing end-of-the-road feeling. He is vulnerable wherever, originally, he had high hopes for himself, wherever he feels he has fallen short of his own expectations.

Once a man starts feeling 'I cannot achieve what I hoped to achieve; it's too late', he is in the grip of menopausal apprehension, and in need of reorientating his life. The death of the dreams can invade all the areas of a man's life: personal attainment, sexual life, marital life, working life, social life. Originally they all combined into a concept of personal significance. It is the fading of this pattern of hope that is often a disturbing feature of the male menopause. Whatever a man identifies as a part of his personal sense of significance may or may not be vulnerable to increasing age. What is vulnerable provides the content for his menopausal crisis.

One of the reasons that women get hit by the menopause psychologically, as distinct from physically, is that they may associate their value as a person too much with the child-bearing role. When their child-bearing role is switched off, they themselves feel switched off. But if they have incorporated the child-bearing role into their lives as just *part* of being a person, then no longer being fertile will not be as profound a jolt as it is to women who value themselves solely in terms of that role. Similarly with men who have placed too much importance on one or other aspect of 'success'.

It is important to differentiate here between the Bond-style extrovert tycoon and the less successful man. The former not only radiates success, but he sets up girls by the poolside and cashes in on his power and position to impress them. That is a very different pattern of behaviour from the middle management type who realises that he's going no further and that it is the end of the road unless he does something dramatic. For the young, the future is a great stretch of exciting possibility, but for the person who gets caught up in the psychological menopause much of the excitement has gone out of life and the future looks like a dreary drift towards death. There is a desperate effort to put something into the void. Then comes the idea that everything was all right 'when I was young' — so they must try to be young again. They must let young people know that they are there.

Counteracting the menopause is not easy. Menopausal men certainly won't succeed by saying, 'I mustn't go around flirting with young girls,' because that's only the surface of it all. They have to start with a basic reorientation of their lives and to accept that life is one continuous rhythm and that as physical powers decline — for example, you can't run up a hill as fast as you used to — then the qualitative psychological side of experience should be developed. Most menopausal men have a bit of catching up to do on maturity. Suppose, for example, a man used to be the tennis club champion and now he finds himself beaten by a fifteen year old boy who has left him puffing hard and with his varicose veins standing out, what does he do? The immature attitude would be, 'My goodness; I've been beaten 6-0 by a fifteen year old. I must have looked a fool.' The mature attitude would be, 'What a splendid youngster. I'm glad this club can attract his type.'

Many people live such a catch-as-catch-can sort of life that they don't develop much as people. They get into the routine of office, home and whatever, and go on year after year without much personal development. Then you end up with a man in his middle years who doesn't know where he is or what he is. That sort of person really needs to start developing those bits of himself that he's neglected and to see the future not as a retreat and a defeat but as an opportunity for the exploration of himself. 'Youth once gone is gone. Deeds let escape are never to be done,' said Robert Browning — but he took up clay modelling in his later middle age. I'm not saying that tatting is the answer to the menopausal phase, but expansion is. Any man of 40 manifests a *small* group of often over-developed potentialities and a big area of under-developed potentialities, and his future lies in developing some of those. The attitude should not be, 'Oh dear, I can't any more to X, Y, Z,' but 'Now I am ready to try A, B, C.' The feeling that time is running out needs to be replaced by a positive orientation that is adventurous and exploratory.

I know a man in his late 70's who even now has shown little sign of being menopausal. He had never travelled far until he retired, owing to other pressures in his life. He could have said, 'Oh dear, I'm getting a bit rheumatic and too much travel can be exhausting.' Not a bit of it. He started to travel abroad, not hectically, but widely, and enjoyed it enormously. He wasn't just hollow inside trying to bolster himself artificially; he was living in the here-and-now and capable of being interested in, and excited by, sights, scenes, and customs that he came across. A man in the grip of menopausal uncertainty would be more likely to go to Le Touquet in the hope of setting up a few affaires.

A menopausal man will probably need some help in reorientating himself and, tragically, it may be that his wife and family cannot help, since your menopausal man is often reacting against too much respectability and conformity and, usually, his family is the source of all that. Or the crisis may come just when the children are becoming independent and leaving home. A good friend can help, but not by saying, 'Come on, you're making a fool of yourself, old man.' Nobody is helped by being diminished — this is Rule One in life, and one of the reasons why I don't like this phrase 'male menopause' too much, since wives can hurl it at husbands to put them down, and that won't help anybody. A man who is at the stage of asking himself forlornly 'Where is my youth?' will probably be best helped by an understanding woman who can gently awaken him to an awareness of his real worth and show him that, by assessing himself exclusively in sexual terms, he is missing all kinds of valuable possibilities in himself. A relationship with such a woman, who may or who may not be his wife, can help him to see himself in the here-and-now and stop searching for things past that are either no longer attainable or only attainable as shams. Our menopausal man may want to wear a psyche that is too young for him. The guidance of a friend can be very effective in getting him to put on a mature psyche. Such a relationship would give him a boost at the same time as it gave him insight.

The relationship, if with a woman friend, may or may not become physical. If the woman has a real understanding of what is happening to the man, she will not let their relationship become sex-absorbed since that would merely take him back to square one. She would use the relationship to broaden and develop him, and so rescue him from the great question mark he has erected above his masculinity, his virility and his identity. In order to be really effective the relationship has to be close and trusting, but an affaire as such is not the answer. The important aspect is the relationship with a mature woman that will give him insight and a new sense of self-respect. This relationship *may* include a sexual component. It depends on the circumstances.

For example, the man may be involved in a marriage which has been threadbare for years. The partnership may have been a mischoice at the start and always without richness, and get to the point where the thin-ness becomes intolerable and the menopausal protest takes over. Many men who are caught in that sort of marital degeneration get crucified when it comes to the crunch because it was part of their dream to be successful husbands and fathers so they cannot easily face divorce. This situation, of course, can happen the other way round — with the woman seeking to escape from a dead marriage.

A good relationship with another woman may become so significant to a man that his current marriage and way of life seem futile. Then, to set himself free to establish a more significant relationship may be very productive. But to break up his marriage in a womanising mood will be self-destructive because he will womanise himself to pieces. You may be able to play the love game lightly when you are young, but when you are older you really *need* profounder relationships. Of course, if the man's attitude to women has always been shallow or arrogant, then he will hardly attract the sort of woman who can be his salvation. He will cut himself off from the relationship before it even gets started.

It is never easy for a man in the menopausal situation, but if he is sufficiently mature to be conscious that something is wrong he may be able to do some life engineering for himself by deliberately presenting himself with fresh interests and fresh challenges. Some recommend a change of job or residence as a source of stimulus and freshness — this can be a revivifying experience at any age. But you have to look at the support system the man needs. Consider a middle-aged man with a reasonably good handicap at golf who plays quite an active part in the club. If he leaves the district to escape from what seems to have become an unrewarding life, he's got to start from the beginning again and, if the club was an important part of his support system, then instead of getting a revitalized personality as a result of the change he may become isolated and depressed. It comes back to the personal equation: if the man is capable of withstanding the jolts, then the challenges and changes can do nothing but good. But the argument is circular since this kind of switch needs some maturity and courage and usually the man with well-developed maturity and courage isn't going to be in the jam in the first place. The people who accept change easily and go around looking for new ideas and opportunities for exploration in life are unlikely to become victims of the menopausal crisis.

The classic menopausal type is the conformist who takes on society's ideas and values without question. When he finds he can't live up to those ideas and ideals, or they lose their meaning for him because they're not his own, he feels himself to be an outcast and a failure. The competitive rat race generates menopausal problems because it is so uninspiring in its ultimate objectives. You don't find the menopausal syndrome getting out of hand when the whole of life is rich and demanding; you don't seem to get it in simpler societies because age, as such, is valued. But although the rat race tends to produce menopausal problems you don't solve them by just jumping out of the race. You may find yourself feeling so strange out there that you may not be able to take it. It all comes back to the question of identity. If an individual has a well-established sense of identity, he can take it anywhere and make something of whatever is there. But if his identity is not very clearly defined, it may collapse when his habitual support system is taken away.

To be in the rat race life paves the way for menopausal problems because the 'good Company man' is work obsessed, and the demands of the job often mean that the man switches his social life from his home to the business area so that home becomes just somewhere to sleep in the evenings and sex is just a little bit of a cuddle when you're not too tired. This gradual deadening of marital life is likely to lead to a protest explosion, which is grossly unfair to the wife — the husband lets his home relationships shrivel and then seeks excitement elsewhere because home seems dull. If a man has lived a tolerable but unstimulating marital life, with his deep physical and emotional needs forced into a secondary role, he is a suitable candidate for the menopausal explosion — an explosion which is the protest of the psyche against an unlived life combined with the anxiety that he will never live that life now.

Often menopausal anxiety is exacerbated by the sound of the pounding feet of the younger men coming up behind. The feeling of being pursued by the young is one of the factors that leads to a sense of the end of the road, and it can take a great effort to readjust to it. The person who wants to be at the top of the tree but who isn't going to get there has to say to himself, 'Life isn't about getting to the tops of trees. Life is about being me and enjoying it.' In any case, getting to the tops of trees is not particularly satisfactory because when you are at the top you are still the same old you. The rat race philosophy overlooks the fact that success and fulfilment are not the same thing — and it needs a pretty big rethink before that truth sinks in. Sometimes professional therapy can help in the personal re-assessment, and sometimes books. Then there are encounter groups, re-evaluation counselling, transactional analysis, and other therapeutic groups. In general, I would expect the kind of man we have been considering to get more help from such informal groups than from long term analysis. But he could well be helped by talking things over with people from one of the auxiliary counselling services such as Marriage Guidance. He would need to go to a psychiatrist only if his difficulties become so dominant that he feels them passing out of his control. For the most part, the menopausal stage is an aspect of personal experience that is best handled by deepened personal understanding.

What the menopausal man needs to learn more than anything is that you only get fullness out of life by living it as yourself, and appropriately to your age. It's no good lying on your back and screaming when annoyed if you are 45, although it is appropriate for a young child. It may well be appropriate for a 6th former to go to a party and cuddle all the girls but, if a 45-year-old does it, he becomes an object of ridicule. The key to discovering what is appropriate behaviour is to accept reality, to accept yourself, to make the best of yourself, to admit yourself. If you pretend to be what you aren't, you cut yourself off from making fruitful relationships, which is one of the essential ways of achieving the new orientation. It can be a little risky to wear a hair-piece, for example, because you may constantly be forced into little subterfuges to protect yourself from discovery. Thus, if you go around constantly giving a false impression of yourself you may cut yourself off from precisely what you need to become well-adjusted, namely: close, trusting, intimate relationships with other people. Self-awareness, self-disclosure and rewarding relationships are the best mechanisms with which to prevent, ward off, or cure the male menopause.

These are only a few tentative points about the life crisis we can describe as the male menopause, but they are, perhaps, sufficient to show that the phase should be acknowledged, taken seriously and studied further.

It is not only the 'experts' who can offer affectionate interest and wise comments. Happily, the world contains many people who are ready, able and willing to signal their caring. We are more than sensible of our debt to the writer of the following letter who approached us from an understanding of other people's needs and not at the dictates of his own inadequacies — as do many of the 'do-gooders' and 'helpers' (both amateur and professional) of this world. His unexpurgated letter speaks for itself:

Dear Mr Male Menopause,
If that's what you think you are in, then there's something wrong, even if it's only being forced to face middle age and finding it hard. Now 46 and having come through, I offer the following, which helped me:—
1. Don't look at yourself with the same attitudes you had at 25. I mean, don't see yourself the way you saw older men when you were younger. Look at yourself the way an older man would look at you. In brief, shed the attitudes of a young man.
2. The years roughly 20-40 are those of looking *outwards* at the world, struggling for a place in it, and in the process unconsciously, or consciously, suppressing or denying parts of your nature that may now be forcing themselves on your attention. Give them your attention. Example: you might have had to deny yourself certain pleasures, including that of idleness; certain interests frowned on by society or disruptive or even supposedly worthless or trivial. This is the time to cultivate them, without any guilt or misgivings. You only have one life and it's yours to live.
3. In the same connection, the second phase of adult life is one of looking inwards. If you're the kind of person who is unused to doing so, or has believed it wrong, then it's unsettling — but *natural and necessary*. There's nothing to be afraid of. If you want to lie on your bed for days, weeks or months paralysed by introspection, then go ahead and do it. You won't die.
4. Paralysis, indecision and desire for change, plus lack of sense of direction and often boredom or revulsion against all previous life seem

to be characteristics of the menopause. a. So what? b. accept them. c. they'll work themselves out. Nature is self-regulating. When an upheaval wells up inside, which seems unmanageable, remember that an outcome also wells up inside. So have faith. Your psyche is working on it at this very minute and will find a solution.

5. What you used to think important may not seem so any more. In that case it isn't. Part with it without regret. Get on with some new things. Sort out what is important *now,* and go for it. (See 2. above)

6. When they say 'Life begins at 40', it means that it is only by about 40 that one begins to have the capacity for really genuine self-knowledge, which is what I have been preaching. Once again, you won't die.

7. Have the courage to discard obligations, people or entanglements that are irksome. Going on with them in that frame of mind doesn't help either them or you. In that field, you've done your bit. If you've been carrying the white man's burden without any satisfaction, this is the time to put it down. There'll always be someone else to pick it up. You've done your bit.

8. Ambition is a curse. Achievement comes from the *love* of what you do, *genuine* devotion. The ambitions of the early 20's are mostly shallow and silly.

9. Have you got a sense of humour? Dust it off.

10.   People love us for our faults and for candour. So should we. Come off it, if you're on it.

11.   You have nothing to lose, *ever*.

12.   One of the most important things that helped me was reviving a friendship with an acquaintance of my early 20's, after a gap of twenty years. We helped each other through.

13.   However attractive, lively, sexy or whatever we were when we were young, many more people want us now for *character* than ever did before. There's a whole world of people in their 40s all dying to meet people of their own generation, to make friends on a deeper and more humane level than nature generally allows the young. Get out there. We're all waiting for you.

Sorry if a bit repetitious and hope it's not all entirely irrelevant. Left out sex. There's more sex-plus-affection around after 40 than even Messalina could cope with. If you're married, then I have no thoughts to offer. Best wishes.

It seems to us that the points made in this letter add up to a totally helpful scheme that deserves the title *The Menopausal Man's Guide to Survival and Growth.* They indicate how to put into effective practice the simple art of changing gear in life with an intelligent use of the clutch — and this latter is crucial, since the menopause may be likened to the crashing of the box, failing to find neutral, and a complete inability to free-wheel.

We have already referred to the male menopause as a condition that attracts and justifies the description 'absurd'. The contradictions and the paradoxes, the impossibilities and the incongruities, the masks, the make-up, the costumes and the postures, the confusion and tension between internal reality and external show: all these contribute to a figure who epitomises absurdity — the circus clown, with his surface smile concealing a psyche in the rictus of silent agony and dumb despair.

> "I am the pathetic one
> Who never succeeds in the ring:
>> Afraid of the lions
>>> Out of time with the dance
>>>> Out of tune with the chimpanzee band.
> I am the one the elephants step on
> For me, the wire snaps and the net breaks
>> Snakes poison me
>>> Fire burns me
>>>> Water drowns me
> And the performing poodle urinates at my feet.
> I play to a full house —
> Always;
> Never an empty seat —
> 'Standing Room Only!!'
> And the ringmaster never missing with his whip.
> God — but why!
> There is no circus
> And
> I am not a clown."

We believe that the menopausal man has only to recognise that there is no circus and he is not a clown (or that there is a circus and we are all clowns) for the *absurdity of his condition* to become abundantly clear to him. And this is where others can have most hope of helping him: he will believe at first that he is the absurdity, and it may take some time for him to begin to understand that it is the condition that deserves the name and not the man himself. Reinforcement of this understanding will help remove the stigma and allow him to see failure in a new light: to fail is not a failing, and the only real failure is to see it as such. It is as circular as fear: there is nothing to fear but fear; and it poses the classic problem of the Gordian knot: to cut through with one swift stroke or to tease out with conscientious dexterity?

Most victims of the condition need to perceive the causes of their situation in their past if they are to find salvation. They need to become aware of how their sense of loss, deprivation and inadequacy started years before and it will therefore be of best help to them to tackle the knot turn by turn and twist by twist and so read the messages on the yarn — as clear for them to see as were the messages of the Incas on their *quipus*, on which the past was recorded in complex patterns of knots in strings of wool.

The unravelling will probably show him the stages of development in his psychological past where the weaknesses first were imprinted and, later, reinforced. He will come to see that he has, as James Hemming put it, "some catching up to do" and the following outline of development may offer some useful signposts and starting positions for that long journey.

In his book *Childhood and Society* Erikson suggests that there are eight Stages of Man during each of which the individual displays qualities which demonstrate that his EGO is strong enough to integrate his personal timetable with the structure of social institutions. The eight stages are:

Trust	versus	*Basic Mistrust*
Autonomy	versus	*Shame and Doubt*
Initiative	versus	*Guilt*
Industry	versus	*Inferiority*
Identity	versus	*Role Diffusion*
Intimacy	versus	*Isolation*
Generativity	versus	*Stagnation*
Integrity	versus	*Despair*

Erikson suggests that the 'natural' time scale for these stages moves from the new born infant to old age, with the last 3 corresponding to the prime of life, middle age and old age respectively. Thus, the menopausal man would come into the category, Generativity v Stagnation, and we see this as being an important factor. However, we would suggest that the options are open to man at any age and that the stages are more use if they are taken to refer to personal development not tied to any time scale, so that, for example, our victims may discover that their essential rejigging needs to be in the area of Trust v. Basic Mistrust.

As we have suggested earlier, it is 'all in the head', and since we accept that the old dichotomy of 'mind v. matter' is a total non-starter (mind *being* matter), this attitude subsumes those that stress the importance of organic changes. The male in menopause is having trouble with his self-ratings. The inner forces that move him towards a unified identity and a favourable self-image have come into conflict with those external forces that require him to keep his perceptions in line with what is realistic. It is the way a man balances these forces that will govern how high or low, how appropriate or otherwise, is his self-esteem — and since the reality factor is represented by the evaluations of the man made by other people, it is obviously relevant whether they are *more* or *less* favourable than his own. The menopausal man can fall into either group, and his condition will have come about most probably after a lifetime's effort of carefully considered self-presentation through which he has tried to manipulate other people's evaluations of himself. His crisis occurs when others do not see him in the roles he most cherishes. (For example, he may be respected by his wife and children as a good husband and father, when what he wants is confirmation as a creative and experimental amateur boat-builder; or he may be recognised as a successful wheeler-dealer in his chosen business, when he wants his son to perceive him as a liberal thinker and his daughter to value him as a model sex partner.) Whether his self-esteem is over or under valued by others does not matter (except it is more unpleasant to most of us when it is under) because his behaviour will be absurd and preposterous simply because it is so inappropriate — so out of touch with what others perceive as reality. If he gets feedback that confirms his success in areas that he values, he will feel good and be soundly future orientated. If he gets confirmation that he has not succeeded in areas where he knows it to be true then for certain he will feel bad and be well and truly trapped in the past. If the confirmations vacillate between what he wants and does not want, if he is confirmed in areas where he has no need and disconfirmed in those where his need is greatest, and if there seems to be no unity of self in the diversity of all this feedback — then will he be a first-rate candidate for the male menopause.

The mechanism for prevention and cure is clear and plain — if not easy — and it is all done with mirrors: the three mirrors of self. The menopausal man needs to burnish them all and then steadfastly gaze at the reflections with an unflinching intent. Firstly, to *see* what is there and, secondly, to *do* something about it. His three mirrors are the Physical, the Psychical and the Fraternal. The Physical comes in many varieties from the full-length dressing mirror to the reversible shaving model with one side that magnifies. In this mirror the man needs to check that what he sees is in accord with what he experiences in his body-image, and to take note of what needs to be done (a) to his body, (b) to how he holds it — his posture, and (c) to his clothes and how he wears them.

The Psychical mirror offers the man self-awareness — and he may not be able to focus his reflected image properly without help from a skilled professional like a psychologist, a psychiatrist or a behavioural therapist. It is, however, of crucial importance to his development that he should learn to take some steps by himself. First and foremost among these are a realisation of the significance of *his* observation of his own thoughts, feelings and sensations and the discovery of ways of reporting them (to himself) spontaneously or immediately afterwards.

Some men will find it easier to try this by writing in a journal, but the very act of writing itself is an inhibiting factor because few of us can write quickly enough to keep up with what we are thinking and feeling. A much better method is for the man to use a tape-recorder, and to retire to (say) a bedroom for about thirty minutes every day and talk to himself about what is happening to his heart and head, and then play it back the following day, perhaps just before he does another recording stint. The simple discipline of going into 'retreat' and opening his soul to himself will enable him to explore many parts of his psyche that would otherwise remain hidden. It may seem slightly pretentious at first and the man may have some qualms stemming from self-consciousness, but it is a technique that, if pursued with integrity for a few days, will soon bring rewards of self-knowledge. By externalising his inner experiences to a tape-recorder in such a way, he makes the whole thing concrete — and the reality of forming the words in his mouth and hearing them come back to him in the room will have the tremendous impact that comes from the immediate, the direct and the here-and-now. All in all, it is an excellent combination of being, doing and observing. His personal testimony is both confession and declaration of intent: he nails his colours to the mast — having created the colours himself, built his own mast, climbed up it and nailed them in personally.

The Fraternal mirror is made up of the windows of other people's eyes and they will give him the confirmation or disconfirmation of what he begins to get from the other two. Whereas in the past he may have used their impressions of himself to create a hierarchical system of self-assessment, now he should use them merely to test out what he is learning from this new method of self-observation.

Putting the three reflections together, he will be able to create a three-dimensional portrait which will have nothing in common with the images from his past which were probably cardboard, cliché and con. The new trio of images will give him a set of co-ordinates that will enable him to re-orientate — which is the essence of the exercise.

Appendix

We found that there are so many contrasting views about the female menopause as well as the male version that we decided to include this appendix of material that shows precisely how much speculation and contradiction there still is in this area.

Our first reference comes from Wendy Cooper, author of *No Change* and this extract is taken from a feature for Cosmopolitan in which she outlines the benefits to be obtained from Hormone Replacement Therapy. She is writing exclusively about women.

"In my opinion, behind most apathy lies the conditioned thinking of centuries which decrees that because the menopause is something which happens to *all* women it must be natural and it must be right. If men were the ones who faced atrophy of their sex organs and abrupt decline of hormone levels in early middle-age, I suspect we should hear very much less about it being natural or right.

The International Health Foundation recently carried out the first large study on this subject, questioning 2,000 women between the ages of 46 and 55, in Belgium, Italy, France, West Germany and Great Britain.

Most women admitted fear of the menopause, dreading the psychological upset only slightly less than the physical traumas.

The symptoms most commonly experienced proved to be hot flushes fifty-five percent, tiredness forty-three percent, nervousness forty-one percent, excessive sweating thirty-nine percent, headaches thirty-eight percent, sleeplessness thirty-two percent, depression thirty-percent, irritability twenty-nine percent, pains in joints twenty-five percent, dizziness twenty-four percent and palpitations twenty-four percent.

When a woman does pluck up courage to go to her doctor, the hundreds of letters I receive make it clear that she has a slim chance of getting effective help. The doctor may make her feel she is wasting his time, dismissing her briskly with the words "It's just your age" or "It's just nerves" or "It's all quite natural". As one woman wrote, "Why should only *menopausal* symptoms be considered natural and needing no treatment? Nobody says this about failing eyesight or decaying teeth."

Even if you do manage to convince a doctor that you need help, far too often it takes the form of a prescription for Librium or Valium, Another woman commented on this: "My doctor says it is all quite natural and gives me pain killers for my back and Librium for what he calls my 'bad nerves'. The treatment makes me more tired and irritable and the whole family suffers."

Time and again women emphasise that families, and especially husbands, are indirect victims of the female menopause.

Our second source is a reference volume by Montgomery and Welbourn *Medical and Surgical Endocrinology*. This is how they tackle the subject of the female menopause.

Clinical features

The climacteric usually occurs between the ages of 45 and 50 years, but is sometimes earlier or later. Its duration is variable. Menstruation itself may stop abruptly or may occur irregularly and in diminishing amounts for some months. Occasionally disturbances in ovarian hormone production lead to prolonged and excessive bleeding. In the British Isles the menopause takes place on the average at 48 years of age. Amenorrhoea in a woman under 40 is unlikely to be menopausal, while uterine bleeding after 55 should be regarded as pathological.

The genital organs and breasts atrophy and the skin loses its elasticity. In some women the changes are slight and delayed, probably because of the low output of oestrogens from the ovarian stroma, which continues for some years, and possibly owing to the activity of the adrenals. In most the uterus decreases progressively in size and undergoes fibrous replacement. The vagina atrophies and the loss of glycogen from the cells results in loss of acid from the vaginal secretion. Corroborative evidence of oestrogen deficiency may be found in the regressive changes in the vaginal cytology. This may be the cause of post-menopausal pruritus vulvae.

Metabolic disturbances, related to loss of the anabolic properties of oestrogens, are not uncommon. They include depletion of protein and obesity. Some women tend to gain weight and to develop fat around the abdomen and hips. Atrophy of the skeleton usually accompanies the menopause and may progress to osteoporosis.

Atherosclerosis and hypertension increase in frequency after the climacteric. Up to the age of 45 women are much less susceptible than men to ischaemic heart disease, but by the age of 70 the sex incidence is equal. The cause may be related to the capacity of oestrogens to lower the level of cholesterol in the blood. Diabetes mellitus is commoner after the menopause than before.

Montgomery and Welbourn write of the *Male Climacteric* as follows:

Gonadal function usually wanes gradually with advancing age without causing any untoward symptoms. Sometimes it persists unabated into old age. In some men, however, it ceases abruptly at about the age of 55 to 65 years (or rarely younger). It is thus comparable with the normal female climacteric. The symptoms are loss of libido and impotence, irritability, depression, loss of memory and an inability to concentrate. Hot flushes may occur, but are much less common than they are in women. The clinical features are, therefore, rather vague and may easily be attributed to psychoneurosis. The diagnosis can be confirmed, however, by the finding of a high level of excretion of gonadotrophins (100 MUU or more in 24 hours) or LH, similar to that found in menopausal women. Treatment with androgens is highly effective.

Dr Wendy Greengross does not agree about the hot flushes. Writing for the National Marriage Guidance Council in 1969 in *Sex in the Middle Years*, she puts it this way:

MALE CHANGE
Do men have a menopause?

Men do not have any change such as a woman does at this time of life, but many men undergo a gradual waning of their sexual powers in the 50's or 60's.

As a man gets older, he often finds that all his body functions begin to slow down. Few men have the same energy at 50 or the capacity for physical work as they had when they were in their 20's, and with this gradual slowing down goes a lessening of sexual activity.

Do men get hot flushes?

No.

Do men have abnormal sex feelings at this time?

Some men are very embarrassed to find their sexual desires are awakened temporarily by other women, or even young girls. This may be caused by an enlarged prostate gland which can cause unpleasant natural stimulation.

Isadora Rubin, in *An Analysis of Human Sexual Response* puts forward the Masters and Johnson line:

> It is still a controversial question as to whether or not males go through a physiological readjustment comparable with the female climacteric, or menopause, when there is a sharp decline in the production of hormones. The output of the male hormone (androgen) declines steadily but very slowly in most men until they reach the age of sixty, and remains relatively constant thereafter. Even among octogenarians, individuals with urinary excretion of hormones within the normal range of young adults have been found.
>
> However, some men do show signs and symptoms so similar to the female's that they have been regarded by many physicians as experiencing a climacteric, usually about ten to fifteen years later than in women. One of the symptoms of this may be a sudden *increase* in sexuality — caused by the fear of a loss of potency and the need of the male to demonstrate to himself that he is "still the man he once was."
>
> Where androgen deficiency exists in ageing males, administration of sex hormone may help to restore sexual interest and ability. However, Masters and Johnson note their clinical impression that the obvious elevation of eroticism that may occur after the administration of hormones is not a direct effect of steroid replacement, but rather a secondary result of the obvious improvement in total body economy and of a renewed sense of well-being.

It is interesting to observe how many people place a great stress upon impotence as a shibboleth of the 'male menopause'. Many men and women who wanted to talk to us about the 'mm' syndrome thought that impotence was a sufficient and necessary condition . . . and many used the two ideas synonymously.

Impotence gets another strong mention in *Psychology Made Simple*. The American author comes right out into the open with his sub-heading:

The Male Climacteric.
In the popular mind, 'change of life' is associated only with women. However, the masculine sex also experiences a comparable climacteric period. Few men, and even fewer women, are aware of this fact. Fore-knowledge of the physical and sexual changes that occur in a man at this time of life can save husbands and wives much heartache.

During their climacteric, some men will become irritable, anxious, and restless. Others will experience headaches, heart palpitations, dizziness, sleeplessness, slight forgetfulness, and depression. These symptoms usually pass off with a return to normalcy in a few months. Meanwhile, people will be saying of such a man, usually in his fifties, 'I don't know what's come over him; he's so different.' As in the case of the female, there will be a small percentage who succumb to the irrationality of involutional melancholia.

In his fifties, even the most vigorous male may experience a period of sexual inability that can last from a few months to possibly a year or more. Uninformed wives wrongly accuse their impotent mates of infidelity. This male lapse is usually temporary. It is generally followed by return to sexual virility *and* fertility, unlike the case of the female, who retains her desire but loses the ability to become pregnant (fertility).

No man should feel humiliated or despondent over his lack of virility, or inability to complete the sex act, during his climacteric period. Such inability is a normal occurrence. No artificial forms of restoring or prolonging virility have ever been adopted by the medical profession as a whole. Aphrodisiacs, love potions, and gland grafts are worthless. However, while science has not yet discovered the secret of prolonged sexual power, it does know how to treat the physical and psychological changes that accompany these 'changes of life'. Male and female sex hormones can prevent or alleviate the hot and cold flushes, mental depression, sleeplessness, and irritability of both men and women during their climacterics. Unfortunately, one in two thousand people will become mentally unbalanced despite such treatments.

There is no such 'straight talk' from Dr Bromley, the author of *The Psychology of Human Ageing*. He outlines the mid-life crisis in terms that many people would recognise as an accurate definition of what they believe the 'male menopause' to be and a page or two later seems to dismantle all that he has set up. Here are the two passages:

Presumably we form a more unfavourable impression of ourselves as we grow older. The negative value placed on later ages supports this idea. Aspirations normally exceed achievements, and as long as the individual feels that he still has time, resources and opportunities, he can ignore the discrepancy. Eventually, however, he must realize that the discrepancy is there to stay, and he may blame his 'failure' on himself. One psychodynamic account of ageing suggests that after several juvenile stages of ego development, the young adult either develops an affective and functional relationship of intimacy (usually with a marital partner) or suffers a sense of personal isolation; in middle age the person either becomes generative, i.e. behaviourally and psychologically expanded and future-oriented, or suffers a sense of personal stagnation: the elderly person, finally, either achieves a sense of integrity, i.e. realism, or begins to despair.

This is how he refers to the menopause itself:

There are no reliable biological or behavioural markers for middle age, except perhaps the menopause; but this is not a satisfactory marker, because it is quite variable in terms of chronological age. Post-menopausal women, however, appear to lose some of the protection they enjoyed against coronary artery disease as a consequence of changes in hormone balance. Contrary to popular belief, the menopause is not associated with uniform behavioural consequences such as emotional upsets. The existence of the so-called 'male climacteric' is doubtful, although the notion has been invoked as an explanation for marked changes in the mid-life behaviour of some men.

In *The Male Predicament*, by Dr. Doris Odlum, we come across no overt reference to the 'male menopause' nor the 'climacteric', but the author does refer to a 'watershed' and, neatly turned from an unexpected quarter, 'nature's last kick' or 'the male second adolescence'. Here is her case:

Between the ages of 40 and 45 a man's life reaches what might be termed a watershed. Youth and its hopes and possibilities are behind him. The future stretches ahead somewhat bleak and uninviting with declining physical and mental capacities and the onset of the 'middle-aged spread'. There are fewer prospects for the unskilled worker and, in the case of the skilled worker, especially in the executive and professional classes, ever-increasing competition and more responsibility and stress. It is dangerous for a man to change his job whatever it may be and the skilled worker has little hope of obtaining further promotion.

The family circle is diminishing as the children go away or marry and husband and wife are more dependent on each other for companionship and mutual support. One of the dangers of this time and the later years is that their relationship will become less and less satisfying both physically and psychologically and that their sex lives will have become boring to both, especially to the man. The lack of frank discussion in relation to their sexual attitudes which has already been referred to makes it more and more difficult for them to come together and to bring any feelings of grievance or dissatisfaction into the open. They both tend to conceal them while underneath a sense of resentment only too frequently grows up so that they drift further and further apart.

The menopause is well recognised in women with its physical and psychological disturbances but we are now beginning to realise that an equally disturbing involutional phase occurs in men although it affects them somewhat differently. It is not at all uncommon for men as well as women to develop a depression between the ages of 40 and 55. This is most probably partly physical but may well be reinforced by environmental factors. The wife who does not understand or who is not prepared for this male mid-life crisis may find herself completely at sea in dealing with her husband; as one wife complained, 'He has always been a reliable, satisfied, stable man with a good sense of humour and very conscientious and devoted to me and the children, but lately his whole personality seems to have changed. Now he is moody and resentful and seems quite out of touch. All he does is to grumble and attack everything, our marriage, me, even his job. I just don't know how to cope with him, he is practically impossible to live with.'

It is only recently that we have fully realised the significance of what is now called the male second adolescence. It has been described as nature's last kick. The man intensely resents his fading looks and attraction for the other sex and it appears that he has above all to prove to himself that he can still attract a young and desirable girl. It is well known that the business man commonly fixes his attention on his secretary or typist or some completely undesirable female many years younger than himself, and a similar infatuation is not uncommon in all walks of life. Their behaviour is strongly reminiscent of the way in which they reacted from the ages of 17 to 19. They are as wrong headed and unrealistic as any callow youth and intensely resentful of any criticism or any attempt to reason with them, especially on the part of their wives or friends. Not infrequently they leave their homes and desert their wives, but in many cases it is merely a phase and after two or three years they begin to emerge from their fantasy life and face reality.

A great deal will depend on the attitude that the wife adopts to the situation. The man is completely unreasonable and in many cases prepared to sacrifice his wife, his job and all his future security. If she is in an unstable state herself and going through the menopause, or if the marriage has previously been unsatisfactory, she is likely to react with hysterical outbursts, nagging and jealousy. She may discuss her husband with her friends or even inform his employer. In some cases she demands a separation or starts proceedings for a divorce. On the other hand if she is stable and mature she may treat the situation with understanding or forbearance and if his infatuation diminishes and he begins to see reason the marriage may even be strengthened and their mutual affection and understanding increased.

Generally speaking, the most commonly held views veer to the middle ground of possibility, speculation and requests for more work to be done. Controversy has been rife for some time but little research has been undertaken into a subject that was raised decades ago by the German scientist Kurt Mendel. He called it the 'masculine climacteric' having observed it in a large number of men. He reports that one said to him, "I suddenly find that I am as sensitive as a woman. I burst into tears for any trifle." Another mentioned that he could not bear to read the papers because of the tremendous impact upon him of news of murder or tragic accidents. Another openly confessed that he was afraid to mix with people because he might make a fool of himself by weeping when he was attacked by his nerves. Mendel points out that none of his cases had histories of abnormality and were stable personalities of settled professional routines. Other symptoms reported to Mendel were flushing, giddiness, palpitations, headaches, insomnia at night and somnolence by day. There were also cases of weakening of memory, diminution of interest in the outside world, morbid egotism, neurasthenia and hypochondria. There was also a marked change in the men's attitude to sexual relationships — for some their appetite became totally extinct, but for others there was a dramatic revitalising after the critical period had passed.

Another European scientist, Professor Hollander, studied the problem around the same time and discovered similar symptoms: lassitude, impatience, irritability, lack of confidence, diminution of creative and intellectual faculties, headaches and insomnia.

Dr Hoche, observing similar symptoms however, did not draw the same conclusions. He found it impossible to draw any clear distinction between possible climacteric characteristics and the normal symptoms that heralded old age generally.

Others who have come out in favour of a male climacteric are Havelock Ellis who suggested that it might start in men at age 38 and Marcuse who suggested that it did not occur until between 40 and 55. Kenneth-Walker placed it as late as 55-60. In an article in *New Society* devoted to The Seven Ages of Man, H.V. Dicks of The Tavistock Clinic points out, "The ancient Greeks took 40 as this watershed. C.G. Jung had hinted at a '37 year old crisis'. There is much evidence to support the view that this phase can be as critical a challenge as adolescence — a giving up and a fear of the road ahead."

Professor Vaerting, the physiologist, suggests that the male meno-pause manifests itself with far greater intensity in men than in women. He also dramatically places the greater mortality among men than among women during the critical age, 45-50, to the more violent effect of the climacteric on men. He claims that, "The cessation of the activity of the sexual glands is clearly responsible for the frequency of suicides during the critical age, which is proved by statistical data."

To return, however, to the middle of the road, here is a publication based on the study made by the one-time Scientific Committee of the World Federation for Mental Health, *Men in Middle Life,* by Kenneth

Soddy. Their findings take us back to speculation and the need for enquiry:

The Climacteric

The existence or otherwise of a male climacteric that is homologous with the female climacteric is a very open question, both in stereotype and in objective fact. The prevailing stereotype seems to be that there is no definite climacteric in the male, but this may be no more than an assumption based on the fact that the male has no counterpart to the visible effects of the cessation of ovulation.

There are at present no reliable figures about fall in sperm production with age that can be applied generally to human beings, although the question is considered of sufficient importance to merit investigation in the case of a man in the 40-60 age group, whose younger wife wants to have a child but is failing to conceive . . . Our main point of interest here is whether there is normally a fall in sperm count in man between the ages of 40 and 60, and whether this might have a feedback effect that is at all comparable with the known psychological effects that accompany cessation of ovulation and its concomitants in women.

. . . whatever the appearances may indicate, there is little or no difference between the two sexes in the extent of attitude change, either at puberty or during middle age, that are directly due to hormonal or psychological factors.

The occurrence of depression and the other specific manifestations of anxiety in the middle-age period; or of over compensating behaviour such as over activity and excessive eating and drinking (Wenckebach, Austria, 1916); or of a hypochondriacal shift — giving up drinking and excessive smoking, going to bed earlier, and taking extra care of health; these phenomena also need to be examined further in relation to a possible sexual climacteric in the male.

Dr John Bancroft, Clinical Reader in Psychiatry at Oxford and founder of a psycho-sexual clinic, is about to undertake a series of research studies into the relationships between hormones and behaviour, which he discussed with us in an interview.

My research will cover such areas as the effects of the contraceptive pill and may even look at menopausal man too. At the moment, our understanding of the relationship between hormones and one's behaviour is primitive to say the least. I think people expect things to be too simple in Nature.

There seemed to be quite a lot of literature on the male climacteric in the second part of the 40's and the early 50's, especially the Heller & Myers paper (See Appendix, p.177). It concerned men with *low* testosterone and *high* gonadotrophin levels — but with no other cause for testicular failure. The men tended to experience loss of libido and sexual responsiveness, and attempts were made to counter this by giving them testosterone. Whereas most men with sexual difficulties don't respond to testosterone, these men apparently did — just as you might expect in a straight case of testicular failure.

Now, it was thought at the time that this was not a normal biological ageing process of the testes — comparable with that of the ovaries associated with the female menopause — but a pathological condition affecting only a proportion of males. Nevertheless, they called it the male climacteric.

Interest in this condition seemed to decline until quite recently when a number of studies with modern techniques have examined the function of the testes in the male as he grows older. It now appears that there is an ageing process affecting the testes and resulting in a reduction of hormone production which becomes noticeable from about the 6th decade onwards. This is not a clearcut change, however, and there is considerable variation amongst males in the extent and timing of this. It probably underlies the findings of Heller and Myers but it would be very premature to assume that this sort of ageing process would usually lead to an impairment of sexual function. In some cases it may do and in others it probably does not.

There are different patterns of ageing in men and women and the effects of ageing are also different in the sexual responses of men and women. It's not unusual for a woman to become more sexually responsive after the menopause and it's certainly common for them to remain at their previous responsive state. For a man it is different. He will reach his peak generally in adolescence and show a gradual decline thereafter. There is little evidence to show the decline occurring rather suddenly in a brief period except for occasional cases where there is a pathological condition. It is much more a gradual process, the speed of which will be affected by a variety of factors.

The process will almost certainly be speeded up if there are other problems operating that make sex a difficult issue — and any difficulty with sex can so easily be over-estimated. A lot of men assume they shouldn't expect as much of themselves as they get a bit older. Consequently they do themselves an injustice and perform less well. There is a widespread belief that once you've ejaculated, that's the end of it for that day. Even young men in their 30's no longer expect any further response. True, it won't be so spontaneous after the first orgasm, but that is not to say they will not respond given appropriate stimulation. Too many couples rather spoil their relationship by making that assumption, whereas they could get more out of it if they didn't think, "Oh, that's the end." This is particularly relevant when dealing with a relative increase in the woman's responsiveness at a time when the man's is decreasing. It is quite a common cause of sexual difficulties in a relationship. Kinsey's gross data certainly supports this point of view.

There are many factors that affect the ageing process: changes in family structure, children leaving home, loss of parent figures, threats to self-esteem by physical ageing or work changes. Work is, or has been in the past, very important to a man's self-esteem. All these factors can come together to produce problems in men's lives which one can call mid-life crises, but of course the timing of it is much more varied — and as far as I'm concerned there is no evidence to show that this is predictably associated with any hormonal change, nor to show that it can be usefully described as a menopause.

It's all part of personal development and individual reaction to environment. A man has to come to terms with the fact that his body is not what it was and each individual's response will depend upon how much that has been the basis of his self-esteem. One man may have depended a lot on his good looks and the attention he got from women to make him feel good. Another may have depended upon his sporting ability or his strength. When something happens to undermine these in a serious way — loss of looks or the onset of arthritis — he will undergo the kind of crisis that will not affect a man whose self-esteem was based upon other factors.

There are very few men to whom sex is unimportant although quite often a man will come to terms with being relatively asexual at an early stage in his life. For such a man later changes in sexuality are comparatively unimportant. But the majority of men are traumatically affected by anything that impairs their sexual responsiveness. A common experience is for a man in his mid-life period, the 40's, to experience a relatively trivial sexual failure and to get it all out of proportion. He may have had a bit too much to drink, may have got a bit depressed, or may have been physically ill and, just because he was not so young as he was, he may not have been so responsive. His performance may have been a little impaired, and he may misinterpret this and see it as a terrible disaster. And, of course, there is nothing like the fear of failure to ensure failure in sexual activity. So what should have been a transient episode becomes a big issue and can provoke a real crisis: "My God, I'm getting old. I can't have sex any more. I'm really over the top now."

If a man's sense of masculinity, of being a successful male, is significantly dependent upon his work role and that becomes threatened, he will need to bolster up his self-esteem in other ways. He may well turn to other aspects of himself, such as his sexual performance, to see if that will give him the boost. Now this may throw some strain on to that aspect and he will start to become more conscious of whether he's being sexually successful. On top of all the other problems this could precipitate sexual failure as well and the whole thing would spiral and escalate. Many sexual problems of the male, particularly erectile impotence, are problems of coming to terms with their normal ageing process and throwing up serious anxieties *en route.*

An important medical responsibility is to ensure that, when a patient presents erectile impotence, there is no physical disease underlying it: the commonest example comes with diabetes. While it is important to check for physical causes it is also important to remember that they are not at the root of most cases of male impotence. Even if there is a physical basis, it may be reversible — and the sexual problem may be then maintained by psychological factors. This is often the case with impotence caused by drugs. *Drugs quite often interfere with sexual response* but the problem continues after the drugs have stopped because by that time the man's psyche has taken over.

Although it is not a rarity to have a low testosterone level in impotent men, it is something of a rarity to have a convincing therapeutic response to giving testosterone. In quite a lot of cases one gets a placebo effect. But I had one patient recently, a man of about 50, who had had mumps when he was 35, and his testes had been affected. He had been more or less OK until about a couple of years before and then, presumably because of ageing on top of the damage that had already been done to his testes, he found his sexual response was waning. He responded very dramatically to testosterone. But that sort of case is few and far between.

The thing is that we don't know the answers to these questions really, because the relationship between hormones and behaviour is very unclear. Some studies of impotence or sexual dysfunction in middle age show low levels of testosterone; some show no difference; some show the range to be very wide; and some have shown that the levels are not related to sexual activity. As I say, it is still very unclear.

And now to return to published material . . . and the first extract, about the female menopause, comes from an author who created quite a stir when he first wrote about sex — well over fifty years ago. This is from *Ideal Marriage* by Th. H. Van der Velde M.D., formerly Director of the gynaecological clinic at Haarlem.

As we have seen how immensely the function of the ovaries influences women's chemical processes (metabolism) and psychic states, we shall readily understand that cessation of this function must affect all the activities of the organism. The cyclic ebb and flow of maturity ceases and the vital processes remain at a continuous level, *of a lesser degree of vigour and acuteness than the average of former years.*

One of the signs of changes in metabolism is frequently increased development of fat all over the body. Characteristic symptoms of the days of vital ebb, and menstruation, tend to appear in chronic form. The disturbances of circulation are most trying. They include sudden flushes and "waves of heat," the face becomes suddenly and deeply flushed; perspiration is excessive and sudden, there are palpitations, dizziness, vertigo, roaring in the ears and blackness before the eyes; all the signs of faintness.

The psychic symptoms during the change of life may be not only painful but much more protracted and obstinate — corresponding to their cause — than similar disturbances just before and during the menstrual periods. Caprice, excitability, increased impulsiveness combined with diminished power of reason and reflection, depression with a tendency to melancholia, are all frequent manifestations, though generally remaining within the limits of what is excusable and endurable. But in women who before this stage in their development have had no mental poise or stability of character, in neurotics, in hysterical cases, and those whose heredity shows morbid tendencies — the "change" causes a degree of psychic suffering and storm which is positively *dangerous* to themselves and others.

These climacteric derangements are specially conspicuous when the menses and the function of ovulation both cease abruptly and at one stroke. But when the climacteric proceeds *gradually*, with slowly decreasing menses, at longer intervals — which denotes that the ovarian function stops by slow degrees — the general bodily and particularly mental disturbances are much less pronounced and more easily endured and conquered. Among these gradual climacteric cases we find those individual women who show complete mental and emotional balance and sweet serenity of temper during the critical age.

A Dictionary of Symptoms, by Joan Gomez, Paladin, London, 1970.

The Change of life
The change of life, when the periods cease (the menopause) is the counterpart to adolescence, and its effects are comparable, and as natural. It may pass without noticeable disturbance, or there may be discomforts and even comical effects, but the end of the change is invariably the beginning of a better life, when dignity, tolerance, serenity and assurance, combine with a period of usually untroubled physical health.
Age: The change may occur at any time from 39 to 59 but the average in Britain and the United States is around 47. Symptoms may spread over 1 to 5 years, if present at all.
Identification: 'Hot flushes', comparable to the easy blushing of the 16-year-old: reddening of face and neck, accompanied by sweating and followed by a cold shiver, brought on by nervousness and a hot

atmosphere, but sometimes occurring in bed at night. Headaches, dizzy spells. Moodiness, including depression and crying without much reason, inability to concentrate, grumpiness, loneliness. Variability in appetite, usually an increase. Dyspepsia, flatulence, constipation. Irregular periods, sometimes flooding, sometimes scanty.

None of these disturbances may occur at all, or some may be noticed, not all, and not all the time, but as capriciously as the English weather: one day fine, the next stormy.

Treatment:

1. General: Have a medical check to eliminate any physical troubles. Avoid middle-aged spread by care over diet. To avoid precipitating a hot flush do not take alcohol, coffee, seasoned dishes or very hot baths, and do not go into a hot atmosphere.

2. Medical: Your doctor may prescribe a sedative or a hormone medicine to tide you over a bad patch, but these are not usually necessary.

Avoid self-pity and long discussions of your symptoms: the change is a natural and healthful transition period. For more complete understanding, ask your doctor's advice, or read one of these:

Family Doctor booklet *The Change of Life,* published BMA.

Change of Life: Facts and Fallacies of Middle Age, by Medica, published Delisle.

Woman: Her Change of Life, by Miriam Lincoln, published Williams and Norgate.

Fallacies:

The change does not produce white hair or other signs of ageing. It does not produce a middle-aged spread, unless you eat more, but there is a tendency for the figure to thicken at the waist and shoulders proportionately and for the breasts to become smaller. There is no loss of femininity although the facial hair may become slightly more noticeable. It does not mean the end of sexual desire or intercourse. There may be a temporary diminution in desire, but afterwards sexual life can be very satisfactory, untrammelled by fear of pregnancy.

And now we turn to the much quoted Heller and Myers paper:

THE MALE CLIMACTERIC, ITS SYMPTOMATOLOGY, DIAGNOSIS AND TREATMENT

Use of urinary gonadotropins, therapeutic test with testosterone propionate and testicular biopsies in delineating the male climacteric from psychoneurosis and psychogenic impotence

Carl G. Heller, M.D., Ph.D. Vancouver, Wash. and Gordon B. Myers, M.D., Detroit

During the past few years several articles have been published in medical journals about a syndrome occurring in middle aged men which has been termed the male climacteric. The syndrome has been characterized principally by nervousness, psychic depression, impaired memory, the inability to concentrate, easy fatigability, insomnia, hot flushes, periodic sweating and loss of sexual vigor. The chief basis for the diagnosis of male climacteric in published reports has been the similarity of the symptoms to those of the female menopause and the relief sometimes afforded by androgenic therapy. The claim has been made that most men and all women pass through the climacteric during the fifth decade and that the diagnosis of male climacteric is frequently missed. Quite recently this concept has been popularized by Paul de Druif in the July 1944 issue of *Reader's Digest,* and physicians are deluged with requests for treatment by hopeful readers.

No objective evidence has been brought forward to prove that the male climacteric is an actual clinical entity or to differentiate it conclusively from psychoneurosis or psychogenic impotence. In fact, ordinary clinical experience arouses considerable skepticism as to the existence of the male climacteric because of (a) the similarity between symptoms attributed to this syndrome and those referable to psychoneurosis, (b) the retention of fertility by most men well into old age, (c) the absence of regressive changes in secondary sexual characteristics of most elderly men comparable to those which customarily occur in women after the menopause. In most elderly women there are unmistakable signs of ovarian failure, namely atrophy of the uterus, vagina, external genitalia and breasts, a deepening of the voice, a tendency toward hirsutism and a loss of feminine bodily contours. In contrast, most elderly men exhibit no physical signs of testicular failure: genitalia and secondary sexual characteristics show no regressive changes, beard and bodily hair remain intact, and bodily contours remain masculine. Skepticism towards the existence of the male climacteric is clearly expressed in a recent editorial in *The Journal.*

Our purpose in this communication is to present evidence which will provide answers to the following questions: 1. Is there an organic basis for justifying the claim that the male climacteric is a true clinical entity? 2. Is it possible to distinguish between the male climacteric and psychoneurosis or psychogenic impotence either clinically by laboratory methods or both? 3. If the syndrome exists, what therapy is advisable? 4. Is the male climacteric a normal accompaniment of the ageing process or is it a pathologic problem?

To answer the foregoing questions we needed some objective criterion of testicular function. It seemed likely that the titer of urinary gonadotropins might reflect gonadal function in the male as well as in the female.

An elevation in the titer of gonadotropins excreted in the urine has proved to be an accurate index of ovarian failure. This invariably accompanies the naturally occurring female menopause and follows bilateral oophorectomy within one to four weeks. The elevated titers of urinary gonadotropins persist for the remainder of the patient's life. There is considerable evidence to suggest that the abnormally great excretion of gonadotropins is due to failure of utilization of this hormone by the nonfunctioning ovaries. Therefore it was decided to perform gonadotropic assays in the male.

Before gonadotropic assays could be used for the differentiation between the male climacteric and psychoneurosis, it was necessary to determine whether elevations truly reflected testicular insufficiency. Therefore determinations were made in a series of normal controls ranging from 22 to 98 years of age and in a group of men with known failure of testicular function. The assays were performed in an identical manner on patients complaining of symptoms claimed to be associated with the male climacteric. In addition, microscopic examinations of testicular biopsy specimens was made in some of the cases.

METHODS

Urinary gonadotropic excretion was determined on specimens collected during a twelve hour overnight period. These were concentrated by precipitating the protein gonadotropins with 95 per cent ethyl alcohol, subsequently dialysing off toxic substances and reprecipitating with 95 per cent ethyl alcohol. The final precipitate evolving from this procedure was dissolved in 6 cc. of tap water and injected into an immature (22-24 day old) female albino rat in 1 cc. portions twice daily for three days. The amount of the gonadotropic hormone in the concentrate was determined biologically from the increase in weight of ovaries and uterus at autopsy performed sixteen to twenty-four hours after the last injection was made. It was found expedient to express gonadotropic activity in terms of actual ovarian weights elicited by the concentrate of each twelve hour specimen. Normal ovarian weights for the strain of rats used ranged from 8 to 16.2 mg. and averaged 12 mg.

Histologic technics used on the biopsy specimens of the testes were routine hematoxylin and eosin stains, Masson's trichrome stain and Giemsa's stain.

RESULTS IN MEN WHOSE TESTICULAR FUNCTION HAD BEEN DEFINITELY ESTABLISHED

Urinary gonadotropic titers of 25 normal men are contrasted with those of 12 surgical castrates and 8 functional prepuberal castrates in table 1.

Normal Men. — Among the normals, all decades were represented from the third through the tenth. All the normal men gave histories of normal sexual function and none had symptoms suggestive of the climacteric. The presence of normal testes was confirmed by biopsy in 10 men, 7 of whom were in the sixth decade or beyond. The 17-ketosteroid excretion was considered normal in 12 cases in which this assay was performed. None of the normals excreted sufficient gonadotropins to cause detectable stimulation of the ovaries of the assay rats. This was evident by the fact that the average ovarian weight after injection with concentrates of the urine of the normal men was only 12.3 mg., which is similar to the ovarian weights in uninjected control rats.

Castrated Men. — In contrast, all 12 castrates excreted large amounts of gonadotropins, as shown by the fact that urinary concentrates caused a fivefold increase in the weight of the ovaries of the assay rats. The average ovarian weight of rats injected with concentrates of urine from castrate males was 62.6 mg., as compared with 12.3 mg. for rats injected with concentrates of urine from normal males. The striking increase in ovarian weight was due partly to follicular maturation and partly to corpus luteum formation. This indicated that the urine of castrate men contained excessive quantities of either of two separate gonadotropic hormones, one capable of stimulating the growth of ovarian follicles in the female or seminiferous tubules in the male (follicle stimulating hormone), the other capable of producing luteinization in the female or of stimulating the interstitial cells of the male (luteinizing hormone).

Further evidence for the direct correlation between gonadotropic titers and testicular function was obtained in 6 patients on whom gonadotropic assays were performed before castration and one month or more after castration. The preoperative titers were normal, the average ovarian weight of assay rats being 12 mg. This was interpreted as indicating normal testicular function. Microscopic examination of the ablated testes showed them to have normal structure, which confirmed the impression that these men had normal testicular function preoperatively. The gonadotropic titers after castration were high, the average ovarian weight of assay rats being 58 mg. The elevation of gonadotropins is probably due to failure of utilization by the ablated testes, which normally metabolize this hormone. Therefore the rise of gonadotropins is interpreted as a reflection of testicular failure.

Functional Prepuberal Castration in Men. — Elevated gonadotropins were also observed in cases of spontaneous prepuberal destruction of the testes. This was seen in 8 cases in which operation revealed either the absence or the complete atrophy of the testes associated with wolffian duct derivatives in the scrotum (table 1).

Hyalinization of Seminiferous Tubules and Clumping of Leydig Cells — From a third type of primary failure of the testes we obtained additional corroboration of the fact that when the testis fails, in the absence of pituitary disease, there is always a compensatory rise in urinary gonadotropins. In this syndrome, only recently described by

Table 1. — *Gonadotropic Hormone Titers in Cases of Known and Unknown Testicular Function*

	Clinical Category	No. of Cases	No. of Assays	Ovarian Weight Mg.
Normal controls	Normal males	25	47	12.3
Controls consisting of cases of proved testicular failure	Castrated males	12	30	62.6
	Functional prepuberal castrates *	8	36	86
	Seminiferous tubule failure*	20	74	80.7
Experimental groups	Psychoneurotic males	15	25	13.3
	Male climacterics	23	109	52.8

* All these subjects were proved to have testicular failure by microscopic examination of a testicular biopsy specimen taken in each instance.

Klinefelter, Reifenstein and Albright and by Heller and Nelson, a definite correlation has been established between the hyalinization of the seminiferous tubules, Leydig cell failure and elevated gonadotropins. The elevation of gonadotropins can be seen for 20 of our cases in table 1.

Thus, in every proved case of primary gonadal failure, impaired or absent gonadal function was accompanied by a rise in urinary gonadotropic excretion. The high concentrations of gonadotropins in the urine were in striking contrast to the low titers encountered in normal men of the same age. Therefore it was felt the gonadotropic titer could be safely utilized as a measure of gonadal failure in cases showing symptoms suggestive of the male climacteric.

RESULTS IN MEN WHOSE TESTICULAR FUNCTION WAS UNDER INVESTIGATION

Urinary gonadotropic assays were performed on a series of 38 men, all of whom complained of constitutional and psychic symptoms more or less resembling those of the female menopause. In addition, 32 of the 38 patients complained of impotence. On the basis of the results of the assays, the cases could be sharply subdivided into two groups, designated temporarily as groups A and B.

A. Normal gonadotropic assays were obtained in 15 of the 38 patients. The average assay ovarian weight was 13.3 mg. for this group of 15 and compared very closely with the figure of 12.3 mg., which was the average assay ovarian weight for the 25 normal males. From the fact that the gonadotropic titers of the cases in group A corresponded with those of normal males it was concluded that testicular failure had not occurred.

B. High gonadotropic assays were obtained in 23 of the 38 patients. The titer of each of the 23 cases was unequivocally higher than any titer obtained in the 15 cases in group A or any titer in the 25 normal control cases. The amount of gonadotropic hormone excreted in these 23 cases corresponded closely to that excreted by the castrated controls. The average assay ovarian weight of the 23 cases in group B was 52.8 mg. as compared with 62.6 mg. for the castrated controls and contrasted with 12.3 mg. and 13.3 mg. for the normal controls and the 15 cases in group A, respectively. It was concluded that these 23 men in group B had testicular failure.

Testicular biopsies were performed in 8 of the 23 cases in group B as a check on the reliability of gonadotropic assays in predicting testicular failure. Histologic evidence corroborating the presence of testicular failure was obtained in all 8 cases. In 5 instances the biopsies revealed reduction in size and in activity of the seminiferous tubules and reduction in the size and number of Leydig cells. The latter were abnormal in granulation and lipid content. In 3 cases the biopsy findings simulated those of Klinefelter's syndrome and are described in detail by Nelson.

Therapeutic test was applied in 29 cases, including 9 from group A and 20 from group B. The therapeutic test consisted in an evaluation of the clinical response to testosterone propionate given intramuscularly in doses of 25 mg. five times weekly for two to four weeks.

Results of the Therapeutic Test in the Patients with High Gonadotropins (Group B). — Definite improvement in the symptomatology was noted by the end of the second week in all of the 20 cases treated. Complete abolition of all vasomotor, psychic, constitutional and urinary symptoms (table 2) was accomplished by the end of the third week in 17 of the 20 cases treated. In the remaining 3 cases vasomotor and urinary symptoms were abolished but the psychic and constitutional symptoms persisted despite continuation of treatment for several months and doubling the dosage for brief periods. It was concluded that these three persons were suffering from involutional melancholia. Sexual potency was restored to normal with these doses in all but 2 cases, in 1 of which involutional melancholia was present. With an increase in dosage of testosterone propionate to 50 mg. five times weekly, sexual vigor in both previously refractory cases exceeded that of normal men.

In 14 cases therapy was subsequently withheld for from four to fifteen weeks and in all instances the symptoms returned and sexual potency was again lost. On resumption of the therapy with testosterone propionate, relief from symptoms was again afforded and sexual potency returned. Thus the specificity of therapy was established. To investigate further the possibility that the improvement might have been due to suggestion, placebo injections were administered. Ampules containing

1 cc. of sesame oil, packaged similarly to the original testosterone pro-pionate, were substituted without the patient's knowledge in several cases. No improvement was noted in any case.

   . . . a case is presented to illustrate the abolition of symptoms and restoration of potentia by testosterone propionate, the recurrence of symptoms and loss of potency after discontinuance of therapy, the failure of sesame oil placebo and the subsequent control by resumption of androgenic therapy. The results of the therapeutic test provide con-firmatory evidence that the symptoms and loss of potentia in the group with elevated gonadotropins (group B) were due to testicular failure.

   Results of the Therapeutic Test in the Patients with Normal Gona-dotropins (Group A). — Of the 9 men subjected to the therapeutic test 7 had loss of sexual potency and 8 had some of the other symptoms listed in table 2. In 3 instances there was evanescent improvement in symptomatology noted during the first week of therapy. However, by the end of the second to fourth weeks none of the 9 patients demon-strated any improvement whatever in either the general symptomatology or sexual vigor.

   The result of the therapeutic test in the group with normal gonado-tropins (group A) provide confirmatory evidence that loss of potentia and symptoms in these patients were not due to testicular failure. This conclusion was corroborated by the fact that normal men experience little, if any, increase in sexual potency or in well being by taking the male sex hormone.

   Symptomatology. — By the foregoing objective tests the 38 cases could be sharply separated into two groups: A, consisting of 15 patients having normal testicular function as evidenced by normal gona-dotropic excretion and failure to respond to the therapeutic test; B, con-sisting of 23 patients having testicular failure as evidenced by high gonadotropin output, comparable to castrates, histologic evidence of testicular degeneration and specific response to the therapeutic test.

   Symptoms Encountered in the Group with Testicular Failure. — After the symptoms of the group with elevated gonadotropins were analyzed it was evident that they fell into five categories: (1) vasomotor, (2) psychic, (3) constitutional, (4) urinary and (5) sexual. The various symptoms classified in this manner are listed in table 2.

   The urinary frequency and hesitancy and decrease in size and force of the stream are undoubtedly related to enlargement of the prostate and decreased bladder tonus which accompany testicular failure. The urinary symptoms are relieved by testosterone, in all probability, because of improvement of bladder tonus, not because of any direct effect on the prostate.

   The vasomotor, psychic and constitutional symptoms are identical with those encountered in the female menopause. Of course, no patient exhibited all of the symptoms listed. The most constant symptom was the loss of sexual potency, which was a complaint of all 23 patients. This was usually but not invariably accompanied by loss of libido. Psychic and constitutional symptoms, particularly nervousness and fatigability, were also invariably present. A somewhat less frequent but more characteristic symptom was hot flashes identical with those described by menopausal women. A significant feature from a diagnostic standpoint was the tendency for loss of sexual potency, hot flashes and nervousness to make their appearance concurrently. While the onset was never fulminant, the patient could usually tell the month or season the symptoms began. The etiologic relationship between the symptoms in table 2 and the testicular failure was borne out by the specific relief

Table 2 — *Symptoms According to Categories*

1.	Vasomotor:	hot flashes chilliness sweating palpitations increased pulse rate headache
2.	Psychic:	nervousness irritability insomnia depression self depreciation antisocial tendencies crying spells suicidal tendencies paresthesias pruritus inability to concentrate
3.	Constitutional:	weakness fatigue muscle pains muscle cramps arthralgia anorexia nausea and vomiting abdominal pain constipation weight loss
4.	Urinary:	decreased force decreased size frequency hesitancy
5.	Sexual:	diminution of libido decreased erections

afforded by androgens, the recurrence after cessation of androgenic therapy and unresponsiveness to placebos.

Symptoms Encountered in the Group with Normal Testicular Function. — The majority of the men in group A also complained of loss of potency usually accompanied by psychic and constitutional symptoms resembling those of group B and occasionally by vasomotor and urinary symptoms listed in table 2. A notable difference was the rarity of true hot flashes in group A. Often the symptoms had been present for most of the patient's adult life or occasionally had been very abrupt in onset, coincident with some psychic trauma.

Comment

At the conception of this investigation four questions were postulated. On the basis of the data presented, an attempt will now be made to answer each question.

1. *Is there an organic basis for justifying the claim that the male climacteric is a true clinical entity?* This is answered in the affirmative by the findings of testicular failure in 23 of the patients studied. The objective evidence for the testicular failure consisted of (a) elevation in gonadotropic excretion, comparable quantitatively with that occurring in castrated males and men with primary gonadal failure; (b) histologic signs of testicular atrophy or degeneration in all eight cases subjected to testicular biopsy. The etiologic relationship between the demonstrated testicular failure and the clinical picture was borne out by (a) the resemblance of the symptoms of this group of cases to that of the definitely established pattern of the female menopause, with the addition of occasional urinary symptoms and the invariable association of decrease in sexual potency; (b) the specific restoration of potency and alleviation of the menopausal-like symptoms by applying the therapeutic test of substitution therapy with androgens; (c) the reappearance of symptoms after withdrawal of androgens, and (d) the complete failure of placebos.

It was therefore concluded that these 23 patients were true examples of the male climacteric!

2. *Is it possible to distinguish between the male climacteric and psychoneurosis and psychogenic impotence, either clinically or by laboratory methods?* Presumptive differentiation may be made by a careful history combined with a therapeutic test. For a positive differentiation, however, laboratory tests are necessary. The assay of urinary gonadotropins provided a sharp distinction between known normal and known castrated men and an equally clearcut distinction between group A and the male climacterics (group B). By this means it was established that the climacteric patients had testicular failure and that group A did not.

This was further supported by the failure of the patients in group A to respond to the therapeutic test. It was therefore concluded that the symptoms of the patients in group A were not due to testicular failure and that the probable basis for the symptoms was psychoneurosis or psychogenic impotence!

On the basis of clinical symptomatology alone, a tentative but not an absolute differentiation can be made. The most important diagnostic points are: 1. Character of the symptoms: The symptom complex of the male climacteric corresponded much more closely to the female menopause than did the symptom complex of the average psychoneurotic. Typical hot flashes, identical with those occurring in the female menopause, are strongly suggestive of the male climacteric but occasionally may occur in psychoneurosis. On the other hand the absence of hot flashes by no means excludes the diagnosis of the male climacteric. In fact, this symptom was absent in about 40 per cent of our cases. 2. The mode of onset: The diagnosis of male climacteric is strongly suggested when a past history is obtained of normal sexual function up until a definite month or season, at which time loss of potentia, hot flashes and nervousness appear simultaneously. A diagnosis of psychoneurosis is suggested when the symptoms have been present throughout adult life or are abruptly precipitated by psychic trauma. Often a careful history will uncover the emotional factors responsible for the impotence and symptoms of the neurotic. 3. The therapeutic test will aid in separating the two groups, since the climacterics can be expected to make a striking improvement, whereas the psychoneurotic usually do not show a specific response.

As the study progressed and the differences in the clinical pattern between the climacteric and the psychoneurotic became evident, a large number of the psychoneurotic were eliminated on a clinical basis. This accounts for the fact that 23 of the 38 patients in the series proved to be examples of the male climacteric and that only 15 psychoneurotic patients were investigated by laboratory methods.

3. *What therapy is advisable?* Before instituting treatment it is necessary to establish the diagnosis of the male climacteric and to exclude the following contra-indications to androgens: (1) the presence or suspicion of carcinoma of the prostate in particular and any carcinoma in general, since the steroids have a carcinogenic action; (2) the presence of edema, since testosterone tends to produce sodium, and hence water, retention; (3) any case showing normal testicular function, since testosterone will inhibit spermatogenesis in normal males and may, in addition, cause disuse atrophy of the normal Leydig cells. In this connection we have followed the gonadotropic excretion in a normal man given a long course of testosterone propionate therapy and found that after discontinuance of the androgen the gonadotropins rose to levels corresponding to those following castration. Whether these changes are permanent or not is still uncertain, but it is entirely

possible that ill advised treatment with testosterone may cause permanent sterility.

Therapeutic Test Suggested for Establishing the Diagnosis of Male Climacteric. — In clinical practice laboratory procedures that will positively differentiate climacteric from psychoneurotic patients may not be available. Although the testicular biopsy is a simple surgical procedure, it may not always be feasible. Under such circumstances it may be necessary to resort to the following therapeutic test: Administer 25 mg. of testosterone propionate by intramuscular injection five days weekly for a period of two weeks. Evaluate the clinical status at that time, noting the effect on symptoms and sexual potency. If, at the end of the two week trial of therapy, the patient has shown no improvement, either of two conclusions may be justifiable: (1) The patient does not have the male climacteric or (2) he will need such an excessively large daily dosage of testosterone that treatment is financially unpractical. If the patient does respond it may be necessary to determine whether the improvement is actually due to specific relief of testicular failure or whether it is merely due to suggestion. Withdrawal of therapy until symptoms return and then reinstitution of therapy with placebos may be required to settle the question.

If the diagnosis of the climacteric is positively established by these procedures and the response to the therapeutic test is satisfactory, the minimal dosage for control can next be determined by trial and error. In cases of complete testicular failure, satisfactory control will usually be obtained by administering 25 mg. of testosterone propionate three times weekly. In some cases injection of 25 mg. once a week will suffice. Rarely 10 mg. once or twice weekly may maintain a patient satisfactorily.

In our experience with cases in which a diagnosis of testicular failure has been clearly established, eunuchoids as well as climacteric patients, the use of methyl testosterone has been disappointing both by the oral and by the sublingual routes. The recommended oral dose of four to six times the injection dose was inadequate for satisfactory maintenance. Larger doses often caused nausea and vomiting and were too expensive to be practical. The sublingual use of methyl testosterone, either in solution or in tablet form, is not recommended because it has either been ineffective or has produced undesirable reactions such as burning of the mouth, swelling of the gums, nausea, vomiting, heartburn, weakness of the legs, tinnitus, vertigo and headache.

If more than two intramuscular injections of testosterone propionate is necessary per week for maintenance effects, it is suggested that pellets of free testosterone be implanted subcutaneously in the thighs through a pellet injector. The implantation of 4 to 8 pellets weighing 75 mg. each will provide excellent control for periods of six to ten months.

4. *Can the average male expect to experience the male climacteric?* We believe not. Our conviction comes from observations of gonadotropic excretion in normal males, examination of testicular tissue removed at orchiectomy for carcinoma of the prostate in aged men, the sexual history of elderly normal men and the bodily configuration and physical examination of elderly men. All indicate that both the germinal and the hormonal function of the testes is preserved well into senility in the average man. Reduction of function is admitted, but fairly adequate maintenance occurs in most cases studied. In addition, it should be noted that the male climacteric is not confined to middle and old age but may occur as early as the third decade. The youngest patient in this series of male climacterics was 25 years of age.

Thus we conclude that, whereas in the female the menopause is an invariable and physiologic accompaniment of the aging process, in the male the climacteric is an infrequent and pathologic accompaniment of the aging process.

The demonstration that testicular failure is responsible for the male climacteric, a syndrome whose clinical manifestations are entirely subjective and easily confused with psychoneurosis, establishes an organic basis and physiologic treatment for a small segment of the large field encompassed by the term psychoneurosis.

Summary

The diagnosis of the male climacteric was established in 23 cases by the finding of pronounced elevation in gonadotropic hormone excretion, comparable quantitatively to that occurring in castrates. This was corroborated in all 8 cases subjected to biopsy by histologic evidence of testicular atrophy and degeneration. The diagnosis was further supported in all 20 cases treated by specific response to a therapeutic test with androgens.

A clearcut differentiation of the male climacteric from psychogenic impotence was made by urine gonadotropic assays, which were decidedly elevated in the former group and normal in the latter. A simple therapeutic test is helpful in distinguishing between these two conditions.

The symptomatology of the male climacteric is different from that of psychoneurosis and psychogenic impotence. Satisfactory therapeutic results were obtained by intramuscular injections of testosterone propionate and by implantation of testosterone pellets but not by the oral or sublingual administration of methyl testosterone.

Although the male climacteric may occur as early as the third decade, it is a relatively rare syndrome, probably affecting only a small proportion of men who live into old age.

THE MALE CLIMACTERIC: IS IT AN ENTITY?

By A. W. Spence, M.D., F.R.C.P. Physician, St. Bartholomew's Hospital, London

In Dorland's *Medical Dictionary* the climacteric is defined as "a particular epoch of the ordinary term of life at which the body is believed to undergo a radical change," and the male climacteric as "the phenomena attending the normal decrease in sexual function in the male." In an annotation entitled "The Middle-aged Man," in the *British Medical Journal* (1953), the following statements appear: "Claims have been made, and denied, that there is a rare syndrome properly described as the male climacteric. The symptoms of the presumed syndrome, briefly, are depression, irritability, lack of concentration, palpitation, weakness, and sexual impotence . . . These claims, however, have been refuted by other workers unable to corroborate them. The so-called syndrome, they assert, is a psychiatric illness . . . .No one has described a condition in men with disturbance of hormone secretion as the only symptom of the so-called male climacteric . . . Until an occult deficiency of testicular androgen — provided this can be estimated — is shown to bear a direct causal relation to the multiplicity of symptoms embraced by the term male climacteric, we have no ground for accepting the concept." These statements were repeated in *Prescribers' Notes* (1953), issued by the Ministry of Health. It is my endeavour in this article to demonstrate that the male climacteric exists as a clinical entity.

Female Climacteric

Before the problem of the male climacteric is discussed it is pertinent to refer to the complexities of the female counterpart, the existence of which, so far as I am aware, has not been denied. Although the climacteric is defined in a modern British medical dictionary as "the menopause," this definition needs correction, for the two terms should not be confused. Menopause simply means "cessation of menstruation" brought about by physiological failure of ovarian function. All women have a menopause — if they live long enough — but not all women have symptoms of the climacteric; in fact, many women pass through this period of life with few or no disturbances.

As the critics of the existence of the male climacteric have insisted that its alleged symptoms must be shown to be caused by deficiency of testicular androgen, the cause of the symptoms of the female climacteric must be considered. At the time of the menopause the level of oestrogen in the blood falls as a result of the ovarian changes, and at the same time the titre of gonadotrophin (follicle-stimulating hormone, F.S.H.) rises through removal of the inhibiting influence of oestrogen on the anterior lobe of the pituitary gland. Climacteric symptoms may be directly due to oestrogen deficiency, to excessive gonadotrophin, or to some other factor. The improvement which may be effected by the administration of oestrogen is no proof that oestrogen deficiency is the direct cause of the symptoms, for their amelioration may be due to the fall in the level of gonadotrophin which the administered oestrogen produces. On the other hand, there are observations which suggest that neither of these two factors is responsible — namely: (1) many women do not have climacteric symptoms although their oestrogen level is low and their gonadotrophin titre high; (2) climacteric symptoms may appear before menstruation ceases — that is, when the oestrogen level is within normal limits; and (3) they do not occur in oestrogen deficiency due to hypopituitarism or (4) in ovarian infantilism. In fact, on grounds such as these Pratt (1950) concluded that a hormonal basis alone does not explain the symptoms of the female climacteric.

From this very brief and cursory survey it will be seen that the aetiology of the symptoms of the female climacteric is by no means established and that arguments similar to those brought forward against the existence of the male climacteric, such as those mentioned in the first paragraph of this paper, could well be advanced to deny the existence of the female climacteric.

Male Climacteric

Landau (1951), discussing the concept of the male climacteric, has stated that the period of life during which "climacteric" symptoms are presumed to occur is also the time at which the emotional and intellectual adjustment of the shift from maturity to old age must begin to be made, and that some men at that time develop neurotic reactions such as impotence and general subjective disturbances. This statement is undoubtedly true, and in my experience these patients are not improved by the administration of androgens. However, similar emotional and neurotic upsets occur in menopausal women and are not benefited by the administration of oestrogen, but this is not sound evidence that the female climacteric does not exist.

In discussing the problem of the existence of a male climacteric and whether it is due to or associated with testicular deficiency the following observations should be considered.

(1) Comparison of Symptoms of Male Climacteric with Those of Post-pubertal Castration

In post-pubertal castration libido and potency are generally diminished or absent, but this does not happen in all cases. Similarly, potency and libido may or may not be affected in the male climacteric. After castration has been performed in the adult he may experience hot flushes and sweats and suffer from generalized weakness, lack of mental drive and energy, diminished power of concentration, a sense of inferiority, emotional instability, and fits of depression. The same symptoms occur in the male climacteric. The argument, however, has been produced that in the middle-aged man they are primarily of psychological origin and that any improvement that may be obtained by the administration of testosterone is due to suggestion; yet I have had referred to me by psychiatrists castrated and eunuchoid patients with such symptoms which have disappeared or have been greatly improved with androgen therapy. Should one assume that the improvement in these cases of known testicular deficiency is also the result of suggestion? This is unlikely, although it must be borne in mind that the improvement in these "neurotic" and "psychoneurotic" symptoms may be secondary and due to the attainment of potency (but see (3) below concerning the anabolic action of androgens).

(2) 17-Ketosteroid Excretion

The urinary excretion of 17-ketosteroids is an index of the amount of androgens produced by the Leydig cells of the testicular interstitial tissue and by the adrenal cortex. Because of the production of adrenal androgens it is often impossible by estimation of the urinary 17-ketosteroids alone to distinguish a eunuch from a normal man. Callow *et al.* (1940) found that normal adult men excreted 3.5 to 15 mg. of 17-ketosteroids in 24 hours and that eunuchs excreted 3.1 to 10.9 mg. in 24 hours. By this investigation, therefore, it is difficult to demonstrate androgen deficiency in the male climacteric. However, on the whole in men of middle age the excretion of 17-ketosteroids begins to decline: at the age of 40 the mean is 14 mg. and in old age 3.4 mg. in 24 hours (Dorfman, 1948). Howard *et al.* (1950) observed that in six patients whom they considered to be suffering from the male climacteric the urinary 17-ketosteroids "tended to be low," the values ranging from 3.9 to 10.2 mg. in 24 hours.

(3) Anabolic Action of Androgens

What is often overlooked or not fully appreciated is that in addition to their effect on the sexual organs androgens have a powerful anabolic action. They promote the anabolism of protein and increase muscular bulk and strength: thus are explained the weakness and early fatigue of the eunuch. One does not therefore have to search for a psychological cause to explain these symptoms in the middle-aged man with testicular failure. The effect of androgens on the central nervous system is not yet known. The psychological symptoms which may occur in the eunuch or in the male climacteric may be secondary phenomena resulting from sexual inferiority, or, on the other hand, they may even be primary, arising through deficiency of whatever action testosterone may have on the higher centres. In this connexion it should be noted that the administration of testosterone to women with panhypopituitarism improves their psychological disturbances and gives them a sense of well-being.

(4) Titre of Gonadotrophin

It is well recognized that high levels of F.S.H. of the anterior pituitary gland are present in the urine of men with primary hypogonadism. Heller and Myers (1944) found that in 15 men with psychoneuroses or psychogenic impotence the titre was normal, whereas in 23 men whom they considered to be suffering from the male climacteric the titre was unequivocally higher. Sniffen *et al.* (1951), who have made a careful and extensive study of testicular abnormalities, have stated that it is unusual for elderly men to have raised urinary gonadotrophin, although it is the rule in post-menopausal women, but that some men do suffer from symptoms similar to those experienced by women at the time of the menopause: in these men they found that the urinary gonadotrophin was significantly raised.

McCullagh and Hruby (1949) observed that in cases of severe hypogonadism in the male the titres of urinary F.S.H. were not reduced to normal levels by the administration of testosterone in amounts sufficient to create normal titres of urinary 17-ketosteroids and clinical signs of masculinization. This failure of testosterone to inhibit pituitary activity in doses sufficient to overcome androgen deficiency they cite as evidence in favour of the theory that a second testicular hormone (inhibin) exists normally and that it is this substance which has the power to inhibit the secretion of F.S.H. Howard *et al.* (1950) have also produced evidence in support of the existence of a second testicular hormone, which they prefer to call "X" hormone: thus, in bilateral mumps orchitis the tubules are destroyed and the titre of F.S.H. is raised, while the appearance of the Leydig cells (which secrete testosterone) virilization and excretion of 17-ketosteroids are all normal. These authors have brought forward arguments which suggest that the Sertoli cells are the source of X hormone and that F.S.H. stimulates its production. According to this view it is damage not of the Leydig cells but of the Sertoli cells which causes the increase in titre of F.S.H. These observations lead us to a consideration of testicular histology.

(5) Testicular Histology

Heller and Myers (1944) performed testicular biopsy on 8 of their 23 cases of the male climacteric. In five they found reduction in size and in activity of the seminiferous tubules and reduction in size and number of the Leydig cells of the interstitial tissue, and in three hyaline degeneration of the tubules. Nelson (1948), in cases which he classified as the male climacteric, observed essentially normal seminiferous tubules but decreased numbers of Leydig cells with abnormal cytological characteristics. Howard *et al.* (1950) and Sniffen *et al.* (1951), on the other hand, found normal testicular histology in their patients, although the excretion of F.S.H. was raised in all.

Howard and his colleagues divide the climacteric in both sexes into two stages: (a) compensated, and (b) decompensated. They state: "In the compensated stage there is a tendency to decreased production of one of the gonadal hormones (oestrogen in the female and X hormone in the male); this tendency is met by overproduction of F.S.H. so that the gonadal function remains essentially intact. In the decompensated stage this tendency to gonadal hormone failure is not counterbalanced in spite of increased production of F.S.H., and gonadal failure becomes clinically demonstrable. In the female the compensated stage lasts a very short time; in the male, on the other hand, one seldom meets the decompensated stage. In the compensated stage in the male, therefore, one would anticipate that the Sertoli cells would be normal microscopically, as indeed they appeared to be."

(6) Effect of Treatment

It has been mentioned above that the improvement obtained in the so-called male climacteric by the administration of testosterone has been imputed to suggestion. Heller and Myers (1944), however, have reported that the injection of an inert oil without the patient's knowledge of any substitution resulted in a relapse.

Conclusion

From these observations and from my own clinical experience I find it difficult to deny the existence of the male climacteric. Heller and Myers (1944) have stated that whereas the climacteric in females is a physiological process, in males it is rare and pathological. Bauer (1944) asserted that on these grounds the syndrome should be termed "testicular insufficiency" rather than male climacteric; he maintained that if the term climacteric is used as it should be, to designate the cessation of gonadal activity, then there is little justification for using the term male climacteric, for although the functional activity of the testes declines with advancing years there is no definite age at which they stop functioning as do the ovaries. In this respect it would appear that decline of sexual function in the middle-aged and post-middle-aged man is not denied and that the problem is one of terminology. If we adhere to the definition of climacteric as given at the beginning of this paper I do not understand why application of the term to the male should be abandoned merely because cessation of gonadal activity occurs between the ages of 45 and 55 in women whereas in men it occurs between the ages of 50 and 70 or not at all. Further, why should decline in gonadal activity of elderly men be pathological whereas in elderly women it is physiological? As Abarbanel (1945) has pointed out, the process of ageing can become manifest in various organs at varying times, and just because the testis may be one of the last to succumb does not mean that it has now become the site of a pathological process while a similar state in the ovary is merely physiological.

Summary

It is considered that the male climacteric is a definite clinical entity, for the following reasons: (1) Similar symptoms occasionally occur in post-pubertal castrates and eunuchoids and are improved by androgen therapy. (2) The 17-ketosteroid secretion, while by no means diagnostic of testicular insufficiency, tends to be low. (3) Some of the symptoms can be explained by lack of the anabolic action of testosterone. (4) The urinary excretion of gonadotrophin is raised — indicative of testicular, but not necessarily of androgen, insufficiency. (5) The testicular histology may show structural changes. (6) The symptoms are improved with androgen therapy, but relapse when an inert substance is substituted. (7) Arguments similar to those advanced against the concept of a male climacteric could be raised against the existence of a female climacteric, which, however, has never been questioned.

From: *Ageing and Mental Health — Positive Psychosocial Approaches* by Robert Butler and Myrna Lewis, published by Mosby.

Although the 'empty nest' (when the children have left home) and the menopause do not ordinarily cause serious problems for women (and indeed may bring a sense of freedom and spontaneity) both of these may become over-emphasised. Sexual promiscuity in order to prove youth and attractiveness may develop as well as increased religiosity that has a hollow and desperate ring to it. Men may be haunted by a need to succeed. All of these represent unsolved fears of ageing and attempts to deny it by turning back the clock. One can see fixation, rigidity, fatalism, pessimism or over-excessiveness. Middle age can be and is for most people the prime of life. But it can be complicated by periods of genuine crisis ranging from the superficial and reversible to the profound and more pathological.

From: *The Ageless Woman* by Sherwin A Kaufman M.D., published by Prentice-Hall, New York, 1967.

Men of course have no menopause, that is, the cessation of the menses. But some men go through a transitional change. This is not the result of any hormonal deficiency. The main change involves their thinking habits — worrying about unfulfilled ambitions, wondering about a waning sex drive, and worrying about their menopausal wives. Such emotional changes are no more pathological than similar emotional changes in the female. The forties and fifties are a time of readjustment for everyone.

Even doctors are not immune. Prompted by a concern for what was aptly termed 'the intellectual menopause', an editorial in a medical journal deplored the fact that some doctors drop out of the world of medicine to escape the pressures of their profession, and urged that the age of maturity is the wrong time to quit.

Just as a woman's libido is not dependant upon her oestrogen output, any loss of sex drive or potency in the ageing male is not the result of diminished hormonal secretion. In both male and female, changes in libido are due more to cerebral factors than to genital ones.

Sources

Bowskill, Derek, *I am the Pathetic One. Circus, Fairground, Zoo,* J. M. Dent and Sons Ltd.
Brecher, Edward, *An Analysis of Human Sexual Response,* André Deutsch
Bromley, Dr. D. B., *Psychology of Human Ageing,* Pelican Books
Butler, Robert, *Ageing and Mental Health,* Mosby, New York
le Carré, John, *A Small Town in Germany,* J. M. Dent and Sons Ltd.
Erikson, E., *Childhood and Society,* W. W. Norton, New York
Geesin, Ron, *Opening for Going Through, Fallables* Pub. Ron Geesin
Gomez, Joan, *A Dictionary of Symptoms,* Centaur Press Ltd.
Greengross, Dr. Wendy, *Sex in the Middle Years,* The National Marriage Guidance Council
Heller and Myers, *The Male Climacteric,* Journal of the American Medical Association
Hopkins, Gerard Manley, *The Leaden Echo,* Penguin Poets. Oxford University Press.
Kaufman, Sherwin A., *The Ageless Woman,* Prentice-Hall, New York
Montgomery and Welbourn, *Medical and Surgical Endocrinology,* Edward Arnold Ltd.
Odlum, Dr. Doris, *The Male Predicament,* The Samaritans
Soddy, Dr. Kenneth, *Men in Middle Life,* Tavistock Publications
Spence, Dr. A. W., *The Male Climacteric – Is it an Entity?* British Medical Journal, June 1954
Sperling, A. P., *Psychology made Simple,* W. H. Allen and Co. Ltd.
Tchekov, A. P., *Ivanov,* Everymans Library No.941, J. M. Dent and Sons Ltd.
Van der Velde, Dr., *Ideal Marriage,* William Heinemann Medical Books Ltd.
Williams, Tennessee, *Sweet Bird of Youth,* Secker and Warburg